Praise for *Calm Your Body, Heal Your Mind*

"*Calm Your Body, Heal Your Mind* is a comprehensive and brilliant exposition on mind-body medicine. The author has done the work of integrating mindfulness and stress medicine in the most complete form I have seen. The techniques presented are excellent and the collated background research is first-rate."

—FREDERIC LUSKIN, PhD, author of *Forgive for Good*

"*Calm Your Body, Heal Your Mind* offers a clear, compassionate roadmap for breaking free from anxiety, intrusive thoughts, and chronic mental pain by addressing their true driver: a nervous system stuck in threat mode. Hanscom shows how restoring physiological safety, rather than fighting thoughts, allows the mind to settle naturally—often after years of struggle. The result is a book that is both deeply validating and genuinely liberating."

—MATTHEW LEDERMAN, MD, *New York Times* best-selling coauthor of *The Forks Over Knives Plan*; cofounder, ConnectionDocs

"David Hanscom is a hero, and in this book, he shares a true 'hero's journey.' For decades, Dr. Hanscom changed lives as a skilled surgeon. Yet it is his relentless quest to understand chronic pain and help his patients overcome it that sets his story apart. Through personal experiences and profound insights, with humility and without self-pity, Dr. Hanscom offers a novel perspective on the human experience."

—C. SUE CARTER, PhD, distinguished research professor; director emerita, Kinsey Institute; professor of psychology, University of Virginia

"This is a brilliant, upbeat, and often riveting read. Dr. Hanscom artfully weaves the latest findings from neuroscience with some surprising findings from psychology, along with advice taken from that most neglected field called common sense. Adding to the book's power and credibility is the personal story Dr. Hanscom tells, which is not only helpful but gripping. Highly recommended!"

—**Edward Hallowell**, MD, *New York Times* best-selling coauthor of *Driven to Distraction* and *ADHD 2.0*

"There is no 'yellow brick road' to curing chronic mental pain, but Dr. Hanscom's new book, *Calm Your Body, Heal Your Mind*, is a great start. His road map is paved with originality, research, logic, and the story of how he transcended his own personal abyss. Beginning with repetitive unwanted thoughts (RUTs), you will learn about the root causes of mental pain and how to manage them. Dr. Hanscom's introduction of tall poppy syndrome and schadenfreude into the milieu offers new and unique bricks for the road."

—**Doug Garland**, MD, author of *The Tall Poppy Syndrome*

"Dr. Hanscom brings to this remarkable book a lifetime of experience not only with surgical successes, but with failures. This has allowed him to look at complex problems from a much wider perspective. He chronicles his journey to explore the intersection of the biological, psychological, and social aspects of pain and illness in a unique fashion. By connecting with the leaders in mind-body science, he brings to the reader a wealth of knowledge that includes genetics, autonomic nervous system physiology, molecular biology, and neuroscience. For anyone interested in new perspectives on health and illness, this book is a must-read."

—**Richard Gevirtz**, PhD, BCB, distinguished professor, Alliant International University, San Diego

"Dr. Hanscom provides solutions for the long-standing problems of ruminative thoughts. He eloquently describes a vast array of solutions through a mixture of scientific and psychological resources. *Calm Your Body, Heal Your Mind* is a compassionate and practical guide to understanding how stress and trauma affect the nervous system. With clear insights and practical exercises, it empowers readers to restore balance, safety, and calm from the inside out."

—**Mel Pohl**, MD, coauthor of *The Pain Antidote*; chief medical officer, The Pointe Malibu Recovery Center

"Dr. David Hanscom has written a book that is both scholarly and accessible. It is filled with scientific information on understanding the role of the brain in pain and in other conditions, and it contains practical methods for coping with repetitive unwanted thoughts. Many will be helped by the wisdom in these pages."

—**Howard Schubiner**, MD, coauthor of *Unlearn Your Pain*; clinical professor, Michigan State University College of Human Medicine

"Backed by scientific research, his personal experiences, and many years of clinical practice, Dr. Hanscom presents a magnificent discussion of the many facets of the human condition and the current distressing human dilemma. If you experience chronic physical, emotional, mental, social, or spiritual pain and suffering (or if you tend to cause this pain and suffering), *Calm Your Body, Heal Your Mind* is an absolute must-read—for the sake of humankind."

—**D.R. Clawson**, MD, physiatrist

"*Calm Your Body, Heal Your Mind* reframes chronic pain with accomplished insight. Dr. David Hanscom reveals pain as a learned threat response; not something to fight, but information to understand. Hanscom is a respected spinal surgeon who has learnt this over years of clinical practice. Grounded in neuroscience and humanity, this book shows how connection, safety, and life engagement restore meaning, freedom, and hope. This book is not just hopeful. It is liberating."

—**Mags Clark-Smith**, MA, pain science specialist; coauthor of *Psychophysiologic Disorders*

"Dr. Hanscom delivers a clear, neuroscience-based approach to healing anxiety, chronic pain, and intrusive thoughts. *Calm Your Body, Heal Your Mind* shifts the focus from managing symptoms to restoring nervous system safety, where real healing occurs. I will be recommending this amazing book to patients."

—**Les Aria**, PhD, chief science officer and cofounder, Menda Health

"*Calm Your Body, Heal Your Mind* is an empowering and accessible guide to uncovering the subtle but deeply ingrained mindsets that quietly undermine resilience, while offering practical, science-backed strategies for everyday life. Rather than minimizing struggle, it helps readers reclaim a sense of agency, peace, and joy even amidst ongoing challenges. An essential companion for those facing chronic physical or mental pain or unexpected adversity, this book ultimately reminds us that meaningful growth and renewed potential remain possible, regardless of circumstances."

—**Brenda Stockdale**, PhD, REACE, CWP,
author of *You Can Beat the Odds*

"*Calm Your Body, Heal Your Mind* is exceptionally helpful and deeply informative. Having worked alongside Dr. Hanscom as a medical colleague for decades, I can attest that he *gets it*, and I quote: 'Consciousness grants us something no other species possesses: the power to choose our response.' Amen!"

—**David J. Tauben**, MD, FACP,
clinical professor emeritus, University of Washington

CALM YOUR BODY, HEAL YOUR MIND

Also by Dr. David Hanscom

Back in Control:
A Surgeon's Roadmap Out of Chronic Pain

Do You Really Need Spine Surgery?
Take Control with a Surgeon's Advice

CALM YOUR BODY, HEAL YOUR MIND

Transcend Pain, Anxiety, Anger, and Repetitive Unwanted Thoughts

DAVID HANSCOM, MD

Foreword by STEPHEN W. PORGES, PHD

Chelsea Green Publishing
White River Junction, Vermont
London, UK

First published in 2026 by Chelsea Green Publishing | PO Box 4529 | White River Junction, VT 05001 | West Wing, Somerset House, Strand | London, WC2R 1LA, UK | www.chelseagreen.com
A Division of Rizzoli International Publications, Inc. | 49 West 27th Street | New York, NY 10001 | www.rizzoliusa.com

Illustration inspired by diagram in Dr. Paul Gilbert's *The Compassionate Mind* (Constable, 2010).

While all the patient stories described in this book are based on true experiences, all of the patient names are pseudonyms, and some details have been changed slightly to protect each individual's privacy.

The information in this book is not intended to be used to diagnose any individual or to treat any particular illness or disease. Neither the author nor the publisher is engaged in rendering professional advice or services to the individual reader. Please consult your health care team before implementing any strategies outlined herein.

Publisher: Charles Miers
Deputy Publisher: Matthew Derr
Project Manager: Elise Menzies
Developmental Editor: Anna Bliss
Copy Editor: Buzz Poole
Proofreader: Laura Jorstad
Indexer: Shana Milkie
Designer: Jenna Richardson

ISBN 978-1-64502-340-1 (paperback) | ISBN 978-1-64502-341-8 (ebook) |
ISBN 978-1-64502-342-5 (audiobook)
Library of Congress Control Number: 2026002462 (print)

Our Commitment to Green Publishing

Chelsea Green sees publishing as a tool for cultural change and ecological stewardship. We strive to align our book manufacturing practices with our editorial mission and to reduce the impact of our business enterprise in the environment. We print our books using vegetable-based inks whenever possible. This book may cost slightly more because it was printed on paper that contains recycled fiber, and we hope you'll agree that it's worth it. *Calm Your Body, Heal Your Mind* was printed on paper supplied by Lake Book Manufacturing that is made of recycled materials and other controlled sources.

Authorized EU representative for product safety and compliance
Mondadori Libri S.p.A. | www.mondadori.it
via Gian Battista Vico 42 | Milan, Italy 20123

MIX
Paper | Supporting responsible forestry
FSC® C103098

Printed in the United States of America.
10 9 8 7 6 5 4 3 2 1 26 27 28 29 30

To my wife, Babs,
who has been there and
supported me from the beginning.

Contents

Foreword

When I first encountered David Hanscom's work, I recognized a kindred inquiry—one grounded in physiology yet animated by compassion. His journey from spine surgeon to advocate for self-healing mirrors a larger transformation in medicine: the recognition that pain, anxiety, and despair are not isolated pathologies but expressions of the body's underlying physiological state. In *Calm Your Body, Heal Your Mind*, Hanscom illuminates what many sense intuitively—that healing begins when the body shifts from defense to safety. His insights offer a bridge between the science of the nervous system and the lived experience of suffering and recovery.

Throughout my career, my research has focused on trauma, development, and the neurophysiology of regulation. I had not thought deeply about chronic pain until David drew me into his community—first through conversations, then through his writings and talks. Though I had not observed his clinical work directly, his insights offered a new lens through which to view suffering. Through his eyes, I came to appreciate that chronic pain is not simply a sensory experience, but a reflection of a body locked in defensive mode. Pain and self-protection share the same neural platform; both experiences are driven by sustained activation of the sympathetic nervous system. When the nervous system remains in threat physiology, the body continues to prepare for injury even in safety, amplifying sensitivity and distress.

Polyvagal Theory provides a framework for understanding this process. Neuroception—the nervous system's implicit detection of safety or danger—continuously influences the regulation of the autonomic state. When cues of threat are perceived, even outside of awareness, physiological resources shift from growth and restoration toward survival. The body's defensive reactions then shape mental experience: Thoughts race, muscles tighten, and perception narrows. Hanscom's language of "threat physiology" and "safety physiology" captures this relationship elegantly, reminding us that healing requires more than insight or willpower—it requires a shift in state.

What moved me most in David's observations was his recognition that patients often became literally pain-free when they felt safe, particularly in coregulated group settings. He described individuals long trapped in intractable pain who, through shared presence and acceptance, began to soften, breathe, and smile. Their relief did not arise from medication or surgery but from the physiology of connection. These transformations exemplify the social engagement system at the heart of Polyvagal Theory: When the body receives cues of belonging, defensive tone subsides, and the biology of survival yields to the biology of healing.

This insight bridged my work on trauma with David's work on pain. Both reflect a nervous system unable to return to a state of safety. Through his Dynamic Healing model, David provides a language and structure that help patients understand their own physiology. He reminds us that we cannot think our way out of defense; healing requires honoring the body's inherent wisdom. His approach—rooted in education, reflection, somatic awareness, and connection—aligns with contemporary neuroscience and restores agency to those who have felt powerless within their own physiology.

Reading this book, I was reminded that safety is not a luxury; it is the foundation of health. Today, many of us live in a world that continually activates our defenses—through digital noise, chronic stress, and social disconnection. The result is widespread dysregulation: inflammation, anxiety, anger, depression, and pain. Yet physiology is plastic. The same systems that encode defense can relearn safety. Every breath, act of kindness, and moment of attuned presence is a signal to the nervous system that the world no longer needs to be feared.

Hanscom's writing is both scientific and deeply human. He translates complex neurophysiological principles into lived experience, offering readers a transformation in perspective along with practical strategies for calming the body and creating new neural pathways. Healing is not the absence of pain; it is the restoration of connection—to our bodies, to others, to life itself. His courage to share his own vulnerability—panic, obsessive thoughts, despair—turns theory into living proof that healing is possible, not because suffering disappears, but because the body, given safety, remembers how to recover.

For clinicians, Hanscom's work reframes health care as a process of coregulation. When medicine treats symptoms without addressing state, it risks reinforcing the very defenses it hopes to resolve. The future of healing will depend on integrating this understanding—that physiology and relationship are inseparable. Safety, in the end, is medicine.

For readers living with pain or anxiety, this book offers a roadmap out of defense and toward safety. For all of us, it offers hope grounded in biology: a reminder that calm is not a spiritual abstraction but an evolutionary design.

David Hanscom has given us a map of the territory between suffering and safety—bridging medicine and meaning, knowledge and compassion. I am honored to introduce this work and grateful for his clarity in translating the complex language of physiology into a guide for healing. May this book remind every reader that safety is well within reach—and it is where the story of healing begins.

—**Stephen W. Porges**, PhD, October 22, 2025

Introduction

The cave you fear to enter holds the treasure you seek.
—**Joseph Campbell**, *A Joseph Campbell Companion: Reflections on the Art of Living*

If you've picked up this book, chances are you know what it feels like when your mind becomes your worst enemy. Perhaps you lie awake at night as the same worrying thoughts circle endlessly: *What if I lose my job? What if something terrible happens to my family? What if I'm not good enough?* Maybe you experience more intense, intrusive thoughts: *What if I hurt someone? What if I'm going crazy? What if I can never escape this mental prison?* Or perhaps your mind replays past mistakes on an endless loop: *Why did I say that? Everyone thinks I'm an idiot. I always mess up everything.*

These repetitive unwanted thoughts—what I call RUTs—affect virtually everyone, but they exist on a vast spectrum. An estimated 95 percent of people have some level of unwanted thoughts, and they interfere with the quality of life for about 70 percent of us.[1] One problem in understanding their prevalence is that many people don't want to admit having them, much less discuss them, because they often feel intensely inappropriate and disruptive when they arise, and tend to worsen over time. My acronym for repetitive unwelcome thoughts—RUTs—highlights the idea that these thoughts can drive our thinking and behavior into a deep rut.

Some people experience occasional ruminations that keep them up at night or distract them during important moments as they go through their day. Others find themselves in the deepest, darkest abyss of destructive thinking, when every waking moment feels like mental torture. You might be a high-functioning professional who appears successful on the outside while battling an internal storm, or someone who has lost nearly everything to the relentless assault of anxious and angry thoughts, or a person caught somewhere between these extremes. Wherever you fall on this spectrum, if you have ever struggled with RUTs, you are in good company.

My Journey into the Abyss

One late evening in 1990, I was driving home to Seattle, Washington, feeling good about the Spine Society meeting I had hosted. I was tired after a long day. As I cruised down the ramp onto the Lake Washington floating bridge, I suddenly began to sweat, and my heart raced uncontrollably. I became light-headed and felt as though I might pass out. Traveling at fifty miles per hour in traffic, I couldn't pull over. For over a mile, I struggled to stay on the road. Then, as mysteriously as they had begun, the symptoms faded. Relieved, though still shaken, I cautiously drove the rest of the way home.

My sense of relief was short-lived. Not knowing what had just happened, or why, was terrifying. Why wouldn't it happen again? Even though I was a physician and an experienced spine surgeon, I had no firsthand experience with anxiety that I recognized and had never even heard of a panic attack. I learned from my internist friend that it is caused by the body experiencing a normal stress response of fight or flight, without an apparent reason.

About six weeks later, on a sunny Saturday afternoon, while relaxing at a college reunion with friends, I experienced another full-blown panic attack. I was grateful not to be in my car but rather at a close friend's home. I spent the next hour upstairs, lying on the hardwood floor of a bedroom. When I re-engaged with my friends, I was fine and told them I had a family matter that needed my attention. Then, another attack struck while I was on the freeway heading back to my hotel.

I discussed the situation with a colleague, and he prescribed Prozac. After taking it for about five days without noticeable effects, I doubled the dose. Chaos ensued as I had a severe adverse reaction. I became so overwhelmed with anxiety that I couldn't sleep for an entire week. That marked the beginning of what I now describe as "the abyss," a prolonged period of unrelenting anxiety, depression, and multiple pain symptoms without the slightest glimmer of hope for an end.

I was thirty-seven years old when I crossed that bridge spanning Lake Washington and experienced the first of many panic attacks. In just one minute, I changed from a fearless, complex-spinal-deformity surgeon into someone battling relentless, growing anxiety along with sixteen other progressively worsening mental and physical symptoms. These included migraines and tension headaches, burning feet, major depression, tinnitus, migratory skin rashes, an itching scalp, heart palpitations, fatigue, back and chest pain, and tendonitis in both my arms and legs. As I struggled to stay functional, I withdrew from my family, friends, and colleagues, and the social isolation became overwhelming. My RUTs had become noticeable during my orthopedic training ten years earlier, but this bridge incident marked an unexpected surge. Of my seventeen symptoms, the RUTs and the social isolation were the worst part. For the next fifteen years, I couldn't escape this downward spiral.

How could I be experiencing so many symptoms? I consulted with many physicians and underwent numerous diagnostic tests. It made no sense, and I found no relief until I finally learned that all these symptoms were originating from a common cause: sustained threat physiology.

The Physiology of Mental Pain

Physiology is a term that describes how the body functions, encompassing factors such as blood pressure, body temperature, sweating, heart rate, digestion, and a wide range of other bodily processes. The body maintains an intricate balance of interconnected systems to function precisely and sustain life and health. Like a finely tuned race car, everything must work in flawless coordination. It takes only a few glitches for the vehicle to malfunction. Like warning lights in a car, the danger signals (symptoms) flashing in your body, if ignored, will eventually result in chronic illness and disease—in other words, dysfunction. The term we'll use for the body being on alert is *threat physiology*.

Imagine a cat stalking through tall grass, every sense alert for predators. The moment it detects a threat—the snap of a twig, an unfamiliar scent—it instantly transforms its entire physiology. Heart rate spikes, muscles tense, and stress hormones flood the system. This is threat physiology, and it's beautiful in its efficiency. The cat either escapes the danger or fights it off; within minutes, it's back to grooming itself peacefully in the sunshine. The threat response has served its purpose and switched off completely.

Our earliest human ancestors operated with the same elegant simplicity. They faced genuine external threats—predators, rival tribes, natural disasters—and their bodies responded appropriately. When the danger passed, they returned to a state of *safety physiology*: rest, digestion, social connection, and healing. But human consciousness came with an unexpected cost. Unlike other animals, we don't simply respond to external threats—we create internal ones through our thoughts. A worried thought about losing your job triggers the same physiological alarm as a saber-toothed tiger charging toward you. Your unconscious brain can't distinguish between a mental and a physical threat. The problem is that while the saber-toothed tiger eventually either catches you or gives up, your worried thoughts can continue indefinitely.

Now consider the stressors of modern life, including career demands, family conflicts, financial pressures, and nonstop news and social media feeds. There is little time for rest in this state of sensory overload. It's no wonder that millions of people are stuck in chronic threat physiology. We're living like cats that can never stop scanning for predators or settle into the restorative peace of safety physiology.

As your brain becomes inflamed, blood flow shifts away from your prefrontal cortex, the thinking and rational part of your brain, to your limbic system, the ancient fear-and-survival center.[2] This is why you can't simply "think your way out" of anxiety or depression. Your physiology has hijacked your higher levels of thinking.

In a state of sustained threat physiology, every cell in the body, including those in the brain, is bathed in stress-related chemicals and responds in its unique way. But why the anxiety and obsessive thoughts? The nervous system is also involved and becomes hyper-reactive. In short, our thoughts are caused by threat physiology, and in turn, the thoughts become a source of threat that we cannot escape. It is a torturous loop.

Everything changed when I discovered the difference between "threat physiology" and "safety physiology." As I learned to regulate my stress response, I became symptom-free and have remained so ever since. I've dedicated my career to helping others achieve the same freedom.

Repetitive Unwanted Thoughts

Repetitive unwanted thoughts (RUTs) are a universal phenomenon arising from the interplay between the conscious and unconscious brains. Since, for most of us, stress is a constant factor of modern life, these thoughts can be unpleasant and persistent.

For example, if a friend hasn't called you back promptly, you might ask yourself, *Did I say something to upset them? Do they like me anymore?* Other situations might prompt you to think, *I am not good enough. No one likes me. I am too thin, tall, short, overweight, ugly, stupid, unathletic, unlikable, unlovable, weak, dull, boring, incapable. I'm a fraud, an imposter, worthless.* Most people feel others have more than they do. This causes fear of missing out (FOMO). These thoughts feel so real and urgent because your body is treating them as actual threats. Then, when we fight them, or try to prove them wrong, we inadvertently reinforce them—a phenomenon that we'll examine more closely in chapter 1. Why don't we have repetitive pleasant thoughts? We don't resist them.

Unwanted thoughts range from mild to intrusive. The duration and severity of your stresses influence their intensity, frequency, and degree of interference. Where do your thoughts fall on this spectrum?

- **Nonissue:** You occasionally notice them, but you are enjoying your life.
- **Irritating:** They are a part of life and don't interfere much with your day-to-day experiences. "I would like to lose some weight." "I wish I had accomplished more."
- **Disruptive:** Perhaps you are upset with someone who did not appreciate you. You feel as though they don't like you. That may or may not be true, but your mind continues to analyze the evidence. Even when you are on a dream vacation, relaxing in the sun, these thoughts keep spinning around.
- **Disturbing:** As their intensity and frequency escalate, they might consume a significant portion of your day, leaving you with less energy to enjoy it. The focus might be on your body image, accomplishments, personality, experiences, or intelligence.
- **Intrusive and invasive:** You have inappropriate, destructive, and bizarre thoughts. They are embarrassing and make you question your sanity. They cannot be suppressed without consequences.

Most people feel that they don't have OCD, and they don't. It is a condition with a lifetime incidence of 2 to 3 percent.[3] Psychological diagnoses have significant overlap, the criteria for specific diagnoses are vague, and there is considerable debate about their value, aside from their use for billing purposes. One research paper has looked at the five most commonly used categories of the Diagnostic and Statistical Manual of Mental Disorders (DSM) mental health coding system: schizophrenia and other psychotic disorders, bipolar and related disorders, depressive disorders, anxiety disorders, and trauma- and stressor-related disorders.[4] This paper also cited other studies. One showed there are almost 24,000 combinations of symptoms for panic disorder in the DSM-5, which is the authoritative diagnostic manual for mental health disorders, and only one for social phobia.[5] The findings of another paper are even more unsettling, in that in the majority of diagnoses in DSM-5, 58 percent of people could receive the same diagnosis and not share any common symptoms. This paper goes into great detail analyzing the problem of creating such specific diagnoses from multiple vague symptoms and perspectives.[6]

Diagnostic mental health diagnoses, in my experience, not only are unhelpful but also cause a lot of damage. When a person is labeled, the diagnosis follows them. Often, they unconsciously live out the diagnosis. It is the reason I will not refer to any mental health diagnoses in this book. That being said, OCD falls under the intrusive and invasive category of ruminations. It is the diagnosis I carried, and it is considered a condition to be managed, not solved. It took me a long time to escape it, and I almost gave up. There is a well-documented link between rumination and suicide.[7] The same concepts that helped me escape this misery can also apply to anyone with less severe manifestations of repetitive thoughts.

From Spinal Surgery to Solving RUTs

There are many extremely stressful professions, with spinal surgery being among the most demanding. The training is long and rigorous, and that is easy compared to dealing with the demands of being in practice. For most of my career as a medical resident and surgeon, I had no idea how to cope with the stress effectively.

I began my career with two years of internal medicine training before I entered my orthopedic residency in Honolulu, Hawaii. I spent six months in an orthopedic trauma fellowship and finished my training at a renowned complex spinal deformity fellowship in Minneapolis, Minnesota. When I began to practice in Seattle in 1986, I instinctively spent time with my patients before and after surgery to optimize the outcome, but I was also aggressive in performing fusions for back pain. During that period, Seattle was performing a high number of spine fusions compared with the rest of the country, and I was enthusiastically a part of it all. In 1993, a published paper showed that the success rate of a spine fusion for resolving lower back pain was less than 30 percent.[8] So, I stopped performing the fusions for back pain, but I did not have effective alternatives. In the meantime, I was spiraling down into my own ordeal of chronic pain.

I tried everything to pull myself out of my misery, and if something seemed to help, I would offer it to my patients and carefully observe what appeared to help them. When I escaped from my multitude of symptoms in 2004, I had little idea of why it all had happened in the first place or how I had escaped. In 2009, I met Dr. Howard Schubiner, who was a pain specialist from Michigan.[9] He was the keynote speaker at a conference I was hosting. As he presented the thirty-three symptoms of Mind Body Syndrome, I counted that I had seventeen of them. My wife and I had met him the evening before the conference. She walked up to him without trying to give me away, and she told him she had a friend with these symptoms. He immediately said, "You mean your husband?"

That was the beginning of solving the complex puzzle, and many concepts snapped into place. I published the first edition of *Back in Control: A Surgeon's Roadmap Out of Chronic Pain* in 2012, and the second edition in 2016.[10] I also created a Back in Control website that presented an organized self-directed healing plan. That is when patients began not only to heal, but to thrive at a level they had not realized was possible.

I began implementing the concepts from *Back in Control* at least three months before every elective surgery. More than a hundred patients with surgical lesions canceled surgery because their pain resolved and remained that way. When I performed surgery, the outcomes were more consistent. It was gratifying to see patients who had felt hopeless and trapped resolve their pain symptoms. I noticed that anxiety would drop along with the physical pain.

My protocol was to have them fill out a detailed intake questionnaire, which provided almost everything I needed to know about their conditions and their living circumstances. I gave them their "homework" of reading

Back in Control and working through the website. A few weeks later, we would meet again and begin the healing process. Not every patient was willing to engage with the material, but most were willing to give it a try. I took the time to get to know these individuals and guide them toward deep healing.

Understanding anxiety and anger was always part of the process, and it took me a while to understand that chronic mental pain and chronic physical pain are closely intertwined. You cannot treat one without the other. The treatment approach is the same: Learn the tools to regulate your body's chemical responses to inputs, shifting from threat to safety. Eventually, I witnessed hundreds of patients become free of pain—physical and mental.

Meanwhile, I was seeing many patients being badly damaged by failed spine surgeries. Often, the effects were devastating. Usually, the first operation was performed for chronic lower back pain from "degenerative disc disease"—in other words, a normally aging spine. Seeing patients heal at minimal financial expense and physical risk compared with the expense and devastation of a failed spine surgery, I decided to quit my clinical practice in 2018 to advocate for data-based healing concepts.

In 2020, I met Dr. Stephen Porges, a pioneer of the Polyvagal Theory,[11] and his wife, Dr. Sue Carter, a prominent researcher in peptides and sex hormones.[12] We formed an informal scientific study group, drawing on insights from thought leaders in clinical and basic science research as well as clinicians from diverse disciplines. Stephen and Sue had numerous connections in many fields, including evolutionary biology, neurophysiology, endocrinology, genetics, and psychology. Their lifetime of relationships with diverse experts facilitated a productive exchange of ideas. We met about twice a month, and the combined knowledge emanating from this group has been groundbreaking. Clinicians involved in patient care have made significant changes to their practices as a result of this dynamic exchange and, in turn, have educated basic science researchers. Many concepts in this book have come from this study group. It still meets regularly, and we are continuing to dig in and refine our knowledge base.

My current efforts operate at the intersection of medicine and mental health, where breakthroughs in our understanding of physiology, neurology, and clinical medicine merge with advances in psychotherapy and behavioral science. I call this approach Dynamic Healing, which addresses the whole person and root causes—not just isolated symptoms. I work with people through a combination of workshops, online programs, and group sessions. I actively teach interested medical professionals and spend a significant amount of time educating the public through various media. Many people find me after years of suffering and ongoing, endless rounds of traditional therapy with minimal improvement. Others have tried every medication available. I have discovered that anyone can heal, regardless of the length of time they have been in pain.

It took me many years as a spine surgeon to realize that many of my patients weren't seeking relief only from physical pain; they were desperate for relief from severe anxiety, depression, and the mental torture of RUTs. I had escaped my own mental prison of anxiety and RUTs and had watched others heal. However, I realized that there were some additional factors involved in addressing these persistent unwanted thoughts.

Many years ago, I worked with a middle-aged woman who had done incredibly well with the healing concepts presented in *Back in Control* and the action plans on my website, www.backincontrol.com. Her diffuse body pain had been resolved, and she resumed an active lifestyle on her farm. I had gotten to know her well and stayed in touch. About five years later, she began experiencing intense, intrusive thoughts, although she did not experience a recurrence of her pain. That motivated me to figure out more about RUTs. Early on, addressing anger seemed to be the tipping point for healing, or remaining in, pain; but I did not comprehend the physiological nature of anger. Nor did I understand RUTs. No matter how hard I tried, I could not help her.

Recently, a young professional contacted me about persistent lower back pain. It quickly came to light that he was suffering from intense, intrusive thoughts. He had been in this state for over fifteen years, and had read numerous self-help books and tried almost everything. His condition kept worsening. Over a period of four months, through multiple conversations and the implementation of the strategies presented in this book, he resolved his RUTs, and years later he continues to thrive. As a licensed social worker and counselor, he had enough medical and psychological knowledge to understand how and why this strategy worked, and his feedback has helped me gain a deeper, more precise understanding of ruminating thoughts. We will revisit his story at the end of the book.

How This Book Is Different

If you're familiar with my previous book, *Back in Control*, you'll notice that while both books address chronic pain, this one focuses specifically on mental and emotional pain, which is often even more debilitating than physical symptoms. I wrote *Back in Control* primarily for people dealing with chronic physical pain. *Calm Your Body, Heal Your Mind* is for anyone whose anxieties and negative thoughts have become a source of suffering.

The healing plan offered here fundamentally differs from other self-help approaches to anxiety and intrusive thoughts: Rather than merely learning to manage or cope with your symptoms, you'll learn to address the root cause of your symptoms, which is the state of your physiology. Instead of fighting your thoughts, you'll learn to change the internal environment that gives rise to them.

Calm Your Body, Heal Your Mind can also serve as a foundation and framework for other therapeutic tools and can be combined with other interventions. Once you have a strong grasp of these concepts, it is easier to choose effective treatments. The solution isn't another coping strategy—it's a transformation of your nervous system that allows for sufficient safety physiology, enabling healing to occur naturally.

Who Is This Book For?

If you ever feel imprisoned by your own thoughts, this book is for you. You might be dealing with:

- anxiety that seems to come from nowhere and everywhere at once
- obsessive thoughts that won't leave you alone
- rumination that keeps you awake at night
- anger that erupts without warning
- depression that feels like a heavy blanket you can't remove
- perfectionism that makes everything feel like a potential disaster
- social anxiety that isolates you from meaningful connections
- panic attacks that make you fear your own body
- intrusive thoughts that make you question your sanity
- any combination of the above

Whether your symptoms are mild or severe, whether you've struggled for months or decades, whether you've tried traditional therapy or medication with limited success, the principles in this book can help you reclaim your mental freedom.

The Path Forward

I've organized this book into four main parts to guide your transformation.

Part One: Defining the Problem will show you how repetitive unwanted thoughts develop and why they persist. You'll discover the science behind threat physiology and safety physiology, and why trying to suppress unwanted thoughts makes them stronger.

Part Two: Stuck in RUTs will teach you about the neurological and physiological mechanisms that can keep you in a mental prison. Understanding them is basic to learning strategies that will ultimately set you free. You'll understand why your body holds the key to healing your mind.

Part Three: Your Healing Journey will guide you through a comprehensive fourfold approach to transcending RUTs and reclaiming your life. Rather than chasing symptoms, you'll learn to transform the underlying conditions that create them. You cannot fight RUTs, but you can "give up" the unwinnable battle and allow your body to heal.

Part Four: Your New Life shows how you can actively create the life you want. The transformational journey isn't always quick or easy, but I've now seen it happen hundreds of times, and I've experienced it myself. The mind that once felt like your greatest enemy can become your most trusted ally. The thoughts that once tormented you can fade into the background noise of a life fully lived.

Your healing journey begins now. Let's take the first step together.

Part One

Defining the Problem

CHAPTER 1

The Curse of Consciousness

The prison is not where you are. The prison is inside your head.

—Unknown

We humans cannot escape our thoughts, especially the unpleasant ones. Unwanted thoughts often appear to arise spontaneously, leading us to question their origin, especially when they are intrusive. Some of these thoughts might feel dangerous or socially unacceptable, such as imagining what might happen if we suddenly swerved into oncoming traffic or confronted our boss in front of coworkers. Occasionally, they manifest as memories, images, or imagined future scenarios and outcomes, causing emotional distress that can be either brief or lasting. Research indicates that they are rarely acted upon.[1]

Recurring thoughts are difficult to navigate. When you encounter an unwanted thought, it's natural to want to suppress it. Why wouldn't you? It's an affront to your value system. Over time, this suppression becomes automatic, a process commonly referred to as "repression."

It seems normal, and what are your other options? The issue is that your nervous system involuntarily gives this random thought more power. You reinforce that neurological circuit every time you suppress a thought. These circuits strengthen and become associated with an increasing number of experiences. Eventually, you might find yourself spending tremendous mental energy dealing with these anxiety-producing, disruptive thoughts. As you feel trapped, frustrated, and angry, your brain becomes inflamed. Chronic thought suppression requires a lot of metabolic energy, which fires up microglia, the first responders, and several other cell types that contribute to the inflammatory cascade.[2]

You are not alone with your hyperactive nervous system. Here are some of the common expressions we use to normalize our chronic stress and RUTs:

"I'm just a worrier."
"That's my monkey mind."
"That's my OCD."
"I've got FOMO."
"I've got imposter syndrome."
"I'm not good enough."
"I'm an adrenaline junkie."
"It's just a midlife crisis."

Almost everyone who comes to me for help with chronic pain symptoms deals with some level of RUTs. It might not be apparent at first because no one wants to admit to them, much less discuss them. These expressions serve to normalize suffering.

Mental and Physical Pain Share Brain Circuits

Imagine you've volunteered to participate in a research study where you're in an MRI that measures activity in various parts of the brain. This type of MRI is called functional magnetic resonance imaging (fMRI). You are playing a game of computerized catch with two other players. The ball bounces back and forth between all three of you—toss, catch, toss, catch. You're relaxed, having fun, and feeling included as part of the team.

Then, without warning, the other two "players" stop throwing you the ball. They continue their game as if you don't exist. You wait. And wait. The ball never comes your way again.

Dr. Naomi Eisenberger led exactly this kind of study, and what happened next surprised the researchers. The brain scans of the volunteers illuminated like a Christmas tree—but not in the areas you'd expect. The regions that ignited with activity were the same ones that activate when you slam your finger in a car door or stub your toe on furniture: Our brains can't distinguish between social rejection and physical pain.

The volunteers didn't just feel "left out." They felt genuine pain. "I feel rejected," they said. "I am worthless." "My feelings are hurt." And here's the kicker: When researchers later subjected them to actual physical pain, they experienced it more intensely than before. Emotional pain had made them hypersensitive to everything.

"Sticks and stones can break my bones, but words will never hurt me." Really? I never understood this as a child. This experiment revealed something profound about human nature: Our thoughts can physiologically hurt us. "You hurt my feelings." "You broke my heart." "That cut deep." "That hit me where it hurts." "I'm shattered." Once you understand this, you'll never view your mental chatter the same way again.

Dr. Eisenberger's paper was published in 2003.[3] Yet the medical world continues to underestimate the effects of thoughts and words on the body, including the brain. Since mental and physical pain are essentially the same entity regarding the way they are processed in the brain, it is almost impossible to have one kind of pain without the other. If you feel you have only physical pain, you might learn that it is actually a manifestation of suppressed thoughts and emotions. If you feel you only have mental pain, consider what physical symptoms you could be ignoring. According to Dr. Eisenberger's paper, you are in a lot of pain either way.

We Survive by Memorizing

Our nervous systems memorize incoming information every second, whether we realize it or not. This is how we evolved. We don't need to continue learning to stay away from a hot stove, avoid a bully, refrain from looking at the sun, or learn how to walk. We cannot unlearn how to talk, read, do math, or cross a street safely. Notice how other animals also retain information. Fifteen years ago, my cat was frightened by the vacuum cleaner used by our house cleaner. Today, my cat still hides in the closet the moment the front door opens and she hears our house cleaner's voice. Animals are motivated by rewards and the avoidance of threats. Humans share these identical drives, with language adding many layers.

Both physical and mental pain are remembered. Riding a bicycle represents a new level of freedom, akin to learning to walk and drive a car. It becomes associated with countless life experiences, both positive and negative. This skill is a permanently embedded set of neurological circuits. I can't unlearn how to ride a bicycle. We can't erase any past experiences from our brain. They become more challenging to retrieve over time, but a word, comment, or image can call up the past.

The Center for Translational Pain Research at Northwestern University in Chicago is a leader in research around the neuroscience of pain. They define chronic physical pain as "an embedded memory that becomes associated with more and more life experiences, and the memory can't be erased."[4] This all sounds incredibly discouraging if you don't understand the solution.

As I mentioned in the introduction, most chronic mental and physical symptoms, illnesses, and diseases share a common root cause: sustained threat physiology, which we will examine more closely in the next chapter. How it works will become clearer as you progress through this book. The dysfunction occurs at the cellular level, down to the level of DNA and mitochondria. The approaches in this book focus on learning to cultivate a safe physiological state, which promotes healing. Everyone heals at their own pace, but the principles are the same for mental and physical pain symptoms. Given my background as a physician and spine surgeon, I will occasionally present cases that demonstrate healing from chronic physical symptoms to show the range of healing that is possible.

No Protection or Escape from Mental Pain

Your body has an automatic protective system known as the nociceptive system, which detects physical pain. The unpleasant feedback signals guide you to act in ways that preserve the structure and function of your body. When the limits of a particular tissue are exceeded, you are compelled to withdraw from the source of discomfort. You reflexively pull your hand away if you feel an electric shock and your body learns to avoid that frayed wire in the future. Although the experience is unpleasant, it is straightforward: Pain signals danger, prompting you to withdraw.

Mental pain is worse. There is no equivalent to a nociceptive pain response. When a disturbing thought arises, there's no physical barrier between you and the source of distress. The idea exists within you, produced by your nervous system. You cannot escape from it or create a physical buffer zone. This absence of natural protective mechanisms makes mental pain uniquely challenging, and for many people, it's far less tolerable than physical discomfort.

In flight-or-fight physiology, our brains become inflamed and hyperreactive. Blood flow shifts from the neocortex—the thinking center—to the limbic system, regions associated with fear and survival. We can't think as clearly when under stress. Our inflamed brain then fires off even more RUTs, which we also perceive as threatening, creating a vicious cycle—like a hamster running on an exercise wheel it can't get off.

The anterior cingulate cortex and the anterior insula, brain regions that process both physical and emotional pain, become hyperactive during episodes of mental distress.[5] Inflammatory markers, such as interleukin-6 and tumor necrosis factor-alpha, increase throughout the brain tissues. There are also microglia cells scattered throughout the brain, which are inflammatory cells. Every neuron in your brain is separated by a space called a synapse.[6] Neurons communicate chemically through molecules called neurotransmitters.

In the resting state, these neurotransmitters are predominantly calming and include gamma-aminobutyric acid (GABA), serotonin, glycine, endorphins, and melatonin. In a threat state, the excitatory neurotransmitters include glutamate, noradrenaline, acetylcholine, histamine, and epinephrine. Some have both inhibitory and excitatory effects, such as dopamine and acetylcholine.

You wouldn't keep your hand over a hot burner. It makes no sense to undergo counseling to understand why the fire is so hot; there is no need to take medications to dull the pain, self-medicate with alcohol or opioids, stop complaining and tough it out, or immerse yourself in other addictive, obsessive activities as distractions. Positive thinking (another method of suppressing pain) wouldn't be effective either. Yet this is often how we approach mental pain. It's absurd.

Dr. Richard Lane, a researcher from the University of Arizona, is a pioneer in the brain imaging of emotion. His group has demonstrated in the lab that physical pain can temporarily reduce emotional pain. People will often choose or create physical pain as an alternative to experiencing mental pain. He developed the Biased Competition Hypothesis, which posits that physical and emotional pain compete for limited cognitive and attentional resources.[7] Survivors of early-life adversity unconsciously prioritize physical pain because it provides a temporary distraction and relief from emotional distress.

I have been perplexed by the practice of self-harm. Self-flagellation, the act of deliberately whipping or harming oneself, has deep and diverse historical roots across multiple cultures and religions. Catholicism, Islam,

Hinduism, Jainism, and Buddhism all have their versions of it. Self-flagellation practices include whipping, using chains or blades, exposure to harsh elements, starvation, prolonged meditation, and severe austerity. Eating disorders and self-cutting, biting, scratching, burning, punching, and hair pulling are modern examples. Neuroscience clearly explains the issue. Externalizing the pain not only offers distraction from mental distress but also provides a sense of validation and control.

We have little to no conscious control over our repetitive unwanted thoughts. Threat physiology drives RUTs, and RUTs, in turn, stimulate physiological responses. Your nervous system is hyper-reactive and responds more quickly to stress, triggering unpleasant danger signals. This is a bidirectional problem with no solution. So, what *can* you do?

Turn down the heat. Neuroinflammation literally heats up your brain, making "turning down the heat" not just a metaphor but a biological necessity.

Understanding why mental pain feels so inescapable becomes even more disturbing when you realize that our attempts to fight it make it stronger. This counterintuitive reality was demonstrated in one of psychology's landmark experiments.

The Ironic Effect: The Polar Bear That Won't Leave

One of the most maddening aspects of human psychology is that the harder we try to control our thoughts and behaviors, the more they control us. Psychologists refer to this as the "ironic effect," which is why positive thinking often fails, why New Year's resolutions usually crumble, and why well-intentioned people frequently suffer the most. Welcome to the two-way trap that keeps us mentally imprisoned.

In 1987, Dr. Daniel Wegner, a psychologist at Harvard, published a paper titled "The Paradoxical Effects of Thought Suppression."[8] The experiment is commonly referred to as "White Bears." It's an experiment that should disturb anyone who has ever tried positive thinking as a solution to negative thoughts. The study employed a between-subjects design with thirty-four participants randomly assigned to two groups that differed only in the order of tasks. Both groups were asked to document all their thoughts for five minutes. The term used to describe this exercise is *stream of consciousness*. They practiced this several times. A research assistant then provided them with specific instructions regarding thoughts of a white bear. Every time they had a "white bear thought," they were instructed to ring a bell or verbalize it:

Group 1: Initial Suppression Group

1. First five minutes; suppression task: Participants were instructed *not* to think of a white bear and ring a bell every time they did think of one.
2. Second five minutes; expression phase: Participants could think of anything they wanted, including white bears, and continued ringing the bell when white bear thoughts occurred.

Group 2: Initial Expression Group

1. First five minutes; expression task: Participants were told to think of a white bear and ring a bell each time.
2. Second five minutes; suppression phase: Participants tried *not* to think of white bears.

The critical finding was the "rebound effect." The sequence of the experiment allowed researchers to compare whether attempting to suppress a thought initially would result in a more frequent occurrence of that thought later, compared with individuals who thought about it normally from the beginning. Participants in the initial suppression condition experienced more thoughts about a white bear during the subsequent expression phase than participants in any other phase did. This result effectively illustrates that attempting to suppress thoughts can paradoxically make them more persistent and intrusive in the long run.

The story becomes worse. Not only did the students think about polar bears constantly, but they thought about them much more than if Wegner had never mentioned them. He called this the "trampoline effect": The harder you push down the thought, the more violently it bounces back. What makes this truly insidious is that the effect doesn't fade over time. It gets stronger. Each attempt to suppress the unwanted thought reinforces the neural circuits. What begins as an occasional intrusion becomes a constant companion.

Sarah, a patient in her forties, discovered this when she noticed a slight imperfection on her face. It was barely visible to others, but once she spotted it, she couldn't look away. "It's ridiculous," she told me. "I know it's nothing, but I check mirrors constantly. I've rearranged my whole day around avoiding certain lighting." Over several months, she couldn't endure it any longer and had a plastic surgeon remove it. Of course, the scar was larger than the imperfection, but somehow it didn't bother her.

What began as a fleeting concern had transformed into a prison. Every effort to dismiss the thought only empowered it further. Her unconscious mind, designed to monitor for threats, had latched on to this perceived flaw and wouldn't let go. The more she tried to avoid thinking about it, the more central it became to her daily experience.

This shows why some of the most beautiful people in the world struggle with severe body-image issues. Their unconscious minds continuously scan for imperfections, and any effort to dismiss these observations only serves to intensify them. Beauty turns into a curse when your mind is wired to identify what's wrong instead of appreciating what's right.

A variation of this phenomenon is the development of obsessive thought patterns surrounding "forbidden activities or topics."[9] Even inadvertent curiosity can stimulate a barrage of thoughts. You cannot "unsee" something. It is also the reason why experiencing or witnessing extreme trauma is so destructive, and often disabling.

The Well-Intentioned Paradox

What is particularly perverse is that the more conscientious you are, the more you suffer from this ironic effect. When a disturbing thought arises that contradicts your values—and it will, because unwanted thoughts are universal—your moral sensitivity kicks into high gear. "I shouldn't think this," you tell yourself. "This isn't who I am." The contrast between your values and your unwanted thoughts feels so jarring that you naturally try to suppress them. But suppression is precisely what empowers these thoughts. This irony becomes even more apparent when you compare conscientious people with those who seem immune to such struggles.

The Trap of Positive Thinking

Most people know about the first half of the ironic effect: Try not to think about something, and you'll think about it more. But there's a second, less recognized trap: When you attempt to focus on something positive, you'll end up thinking about it less. This is why positive affirmations fail so spectacularly.

When you stand in front of a mirror saying, "I am confident and successful," your unconscious mind immediately begins cataloging all the ways you're not confident and successful. It's like having a relentless fact-checker running in the background, constantly undermining your conscious intentions.

Think about your New Year's resolutions. How many have you kept for more than a few weeks? When you declare, "This year I'm going to exercise every day," what happens? Your unconscious mind starts to watch for signs of failure. Miss one day, and it whispers, "See? You can't stick to anything." Skip a second day, and that voice in your mind grows louder: "Why do you even bother trying?"

The research on this topic is both fascinating and depressing. Studies indicate that people who actively seek happiness often become sadder. Those who attempt to avoid prejudiced thoughts might become more prejudiced. The intention to feel better frequently leads to the opposite result.[10]

This explains one of modern life's greatest paradoxes: Many successful people feel like frauds. Despite abundant evidence of their competence, they can't shake the feeling that they're fooling everyone. The harder they try to feel successful, the more their unconscious mind focuses on potential failures. But why does this happen? To understand this, you need to grasp the shocking power imbalance that's been rigging the game against you from the start.

David vs. Goliath

Although we like to believe our actions are guided by deliberate thought, research shows that unconscious processes drive up to 95 percent of human behavior. Our senses flood the brain with up to a billion bits of information per second, but conscious awareness processes only about ten to sixty bits per second.[11] The unconscious brain rapidly filters and interprets this torrent of sensory input, shaping perception, emotion, and decision-making long before we "know" what we're doing.

Conscious thought is slow, effortful, and limited, while unconscious systems operate automatically and efficiently, using emotional cues and prior learning, clarifying ideas through trial and error. As a result, we often act based on how we *feel*, not how we *think*, with emotion-laden, unconscious signals leading behavior and consciousness arriving later to make sense of it all. Additionally, the unconscious brain never stops for a millisecond, whereas your conscious mind can focus on one thing for only a few seconds or minutes. There is both a power and an attention mismatch, and it isn't a fair fight.

When you consciously decide to "think positive" to "focus on gratitude," your unconscious mind immediately scans for everything you should be worried about. Your conscious mind declares, "I am calm and peaceful." Your unconscious mind catalogs every reason you should be anxious.

With chronic pain, there is usually no structural cause for the symptoms. Nonetheless, in my medical practice, I never assumed anything. I consistently had my patients undergo a thorough workup while coordinating these efforts with their primary care physicians. However, even after numerous regular tests demonstrated that there were no significant problems, patients often felt that something was being overlooked. At that point, whenever I spent time reassuring them that they were okay, the reassurances worked against us. They couldn't keep from thinking, "My doctor is missing something because I am in so much pain."

The more conversations we had, the stronger their conviction became. I did not understand that by attempting to reassure patients about their pain, I was helping them to focus on it, further reinforcing these deeply etched patterns in their nervous systems. This is especially unfortunate because it also limits treatment options. The one significant variable that predicts success or failure in treating chronic mental or physical illness is your willingness to engage with the healing process and master the tools. The problem is that these endlessly repeating circuits block openness to learning. This unfair mismatch often played out in front of me in my medical practice. I watched this dynamic hamper many patients' ability to heal, even when effective treatments were available.

Your Demons Are Robots

Those all-consuming thoughts spinning in your head aren't really *you*. They're like robots—automated programs running code written years or decades ago, repeating the same cycles regardless of whether they serve your current needs. As they strengthen over time with repetition, we might begin to think of them as demons.

Not only are they not who you are, but they are the *opposite* of who you are. Otherwise, you wouldn't have suppressed these thoughts in the first place. Eventually, you get worn down. Another consequence of this relentless repetition of unpleasant thoughts is that your body responds with stress chemicals, which affect every cell in your body; after a while, you become ill.

Consider a robot vacuum. It doesn't matter how much you explain that the floor is already clean. It doesn't care about your preferences or heed your reasoning. It simply runs its program: scan, identify debris, clean, repeat. You can't negotiate with it or persuade it to take a different approach. Your unwanted thoughts operate similarly. They are neurological robots, executing patterns embedded in your nervous system. When you attempt to reason with them—"This thought doesn't make sense," "I shouldn't worry about this," "I need to be more positive"—you might as well be having a philosophical discussion with your toaster.

The robots don't respond to logic because they cannot process it. They respond to energy. Every time you engage with an unwanted thought, you're fueling the robot with more power. Each time you analyze why the idea is present, you're becoming more enmeshed in the circuit. It's almost surreal that we dedicate so much time and energy to trying to contain and suppress our demons.

But here's what makes this even more complex: These robots in our heads started as sophisticated survival strategies. To understand this, we need to understand our trauma responses. Some of our most destructive thought patterns began as lifesaving mechanisms that we can't simply think our way out of.

People-Pleasing: A Health Crisis

Dr. Lydia Temoshok is a prominent psychologist in behavioral medicine and psychosocial oncology. She coined the term *Type C Coping Style*. Her discovery should have made headlines. While studying melanoma patients at UC San Francisco, she asked each patient: "When was the last time you felt angry?" The most common response: "I have never felt anger."[12]

This seemed remarkable until she connected patients to physiological monitoring. While they verbally insisted they felt calm, their bodies betrayed them—with elevated heart rates, stress responses, and chronic cortisol elevation. They weren't calm; they'd lost the ability to consciously recognize their emotional states. Dr. Temoshok called this "desynchrony"—the deadly split between what people say they feel and what their bodies experience.

These patients represented the Type C Coping Style. They were the individuals who had spent their lives being the "good" ones: never complaining, never causing trouble, never saying no. They'd learned that survival meant managing everyone else's emotions while ignoring their own.

Think about these common childhood messages: "You can't be hungry—it's not dinnertime"; "Don't say you don't like Uncle Bob"; "Don't be so dramatic." Children face impossible choices: Trust internal signals or trust the authority figure they depend on for survival?

This becomes life's blueprint: Ignore your needs, suppress authentic reactions, prioritize everyone else's comfort. The result? Adults who "never get angry" and always say yes even when they mean no, and their bodies eventually break down under lifelong emotional suppression.

If you've spent your life suppressing genuine responses, your brain becomes overly alert to "unacceptable" reactions. Your internal system acts like a smoke detector going off every time you make toast—except it's detecting thoughts that might threaten your "never get upset" image. All of these patterns—suppression, people-pleasing, the ironic effect—operate like spinning wheels that gain momentum with each revolution. Understanding their impersonal mechanical nature is key to finding a way out.

Stockholm Syndrome or Appeasement?

For decades, psychology textbooks taught us about Stockholm syndrome—the idea that hostages develop emotional bonds with their captors due to psychological weakness. This explanation painted survivors as defective and missed something far more remarkable.[13]

Dr. Stephen Porges, author of *The Polyvagal Theory*, introduced me to the importance of the vagus nerve as the main nerve of the calming parasympathetic nervous system. He defines it as "the longest nerve in the autonomic nervous system, stretching from the brainstem to the colon. It is our internal control center, allowing the brain to monitor and receive information about many of our bodily functions."[14] At the upper end, given its proximity with the facial muscles and the auditory nerves, it transmits signals of safety or danger depending on facial expressions and sounds. Emotions can transmit from one person to another in a process called coregulation. So, if you are angry, you will generally cause the other person to become angry as well. The same is true if you're calm. Your demeanor has a significant impact on those close to you.

Dr. Porges wrote a remarkable paper regarding this situation. What appeared to be "bonding" was actually a sophisticated survival strategy: appeasement. Unlike Stockholm syndrome, appeasement doesn't involve affection. It's a neurobiological survival mechanism allowing some individuals to stay alive by coregulating their captor's nervous system.[15]

When facing an inescapable life threat, certain individuals can access "super social engagement"—an extraordinary hybrid state that simultaneously maintains a genuine social connection with a dangerous person, creates authentic calm that soothes the aggressor, remains internally alert and ready for action, and achieves genuine coregulation between nervous systems.

Think of keeping one foot on the gas pedal (ready for action) while the other gently presses the brake (maintaining calm). Most people's nervous systems can't manage this; they either fight, flee, or shut down completely. This capacity requires incredible nervous system flexibility and biological resources. It's not learned—it appears to be an innate ability some people possess.

Appeasement vs. Fawning

Understanding the difference between appeasement and fawning is crucial because they look similar but represent completely different nervous system states with vastly different outcomes.

Appeasement happens during an actual life threat. It's an unconscious survival mechanism that creates authentic calm in dangerous situations. The person isn't trying to be nice—they're accessing remarkable neurobiological resources that can save their life through genuine coregulation.

Fawning is what happens when that survival strategy becomes stuck "on" long after the danger has passed. It becomes chronic people-pleasing driven by the belief that managing others' emotions is necessary for survival, even in safe situations. "If I am good enough, I won't upset her." You could consider fawning as proactive appeasement.

The progression typically looks like this: A child in a chaotic household learns that survival depends on keeping volatile adults calm. In truly threatening moments, some children discover they can access appeasement—soothing agitated caregivers through genuine nervous system regulation. However, when this child grows up, their nervous system will treat any interpersonal tension as life-threatening. They continue to exhibit fawning behaviors—saying yes when they mean no, managing others' emotions, and prioritizing everyone else's needs—even in safe relationships.

To sum up the key differences between appeasement and fawning, appeasement is a two-way regulation that genuinely calms both parties, time-limited to actual danger; fawning is a one-sided performance that often triggers more aggression from the person being fawned over, and it becomes a chronic social behavior long after the original danger has passed.

People stuck in fawning patterns are especially vulnerable to unwanted thoughts because their internal monitoring system is hypersensitive to any response that might disturb others. Their brains work overtime, suppressing not only unwanted thoughts but also any genuine reaction. This creates ideal conditions for the ironic effect to intensify. The outcome is chronic, simmering resentment stemming from the repeated inability to get your needs met.

It is a tragedy that brilliant survival intelligence becomes a prison. Breaking free requires understanding that these aren't character flaws but survival strategies that have outlived their usefulness. The same nervous system flexibility that enabled appeasement can be redirected, but it requires working with, rather than against, survival priorities.

The Bully Advantage

Meanwhile, people with fewer scruples do not experience this internal conflict as intensely. They might have a politically incorrect thought and shrug it off. They do not waste energy fighting against their minds because they do not take their random thoughts as seriously. This dynamic helps explain why so many aggressive personalities end up in positions of power. They are not as troubled by the ironic effect because they do not judge their thoughts as harshly.

Research shows that anger, self-criticism, and anxiety contribute to increased inflammation and mental chaos. If you are trapped by anything—difficult relationships, lack of opportunity, financial problems, bullying, or RUTs—inflammation increases.[16]

The only caveat is that if you are angry and "win," your inflammatory markers drop. Research indicates that students who experience bullying have higher inflammatory markers compared with those who do not, and that bullies show lower inflammatory markers. This suggests a physiological reward for power and control.[17]

It's a troubling irony: The people our world most needs as leaders—those with deep consciences and a genuine care for others—are often the ones most crippled by their mental struggles. This pattern of conscientiousness creating anxiety becomes most dangerous when it's learned early in life.

Decision Fatigue and the Energy Audit

Marcus was a successful architect who came to see me because he was struggling to make decisions. Simple choices—what to eat for breakfast, which route to take to work—paralyzed him for hours. "I used to design buildings," he said. "Now I can't decide which coffee to order." His story was familiar. It began with a desire to make better choices, to be more mindful and intentional. However, every decision became an opportunity for his monitoring system to catalog potential mistakes. Should he eat eggs or oatmeal? His mind would instantly generate dozens of considerations: nutrition, environmental impact, time constraints, and the complexity of preparation. The more he attempted to make "good" decisions, the more overwhelming those decisions became. His well-intentioned desire for excellence had turned ordinary choices into torture chambers.

This is what the ironic effect does to high-achieving, conscientious people. It weaponizes their values against them. The very qualities that make them excellent—attention to detail, care for others, high standards—become the source of their suffering when filtered through the brain's monitoring system. Marcus's story illustrates a crucial principle: The harder we fight our mental patterns, the more energy they consume.

Your brain is running an energy audit every second of every day, and the numbers don't lie. When you're feeling relatively well rested and not overwhelmed, you can maintain some conscious control over your mental processes. You can redirect your attention, choose your responses, and generally enjoy your life, for a time.

But when you're stressed, tired, or emotionally drained, the monitoring function takes over completely. Your conscious mind, already facing an uphill battle, lacks the energy to compete. Attention automatically shifts to whatever appears most threatening or urgent. This is why RUTs worsen during periods of stress. It's not that you're becoming weaker or less capable—it's that your conscious mind is running on empty while your unconscious monitoring system operates on unlimited power. Understanding this dynamic is crucial because it helps you recognize that the problem isn't psychological weakness. You're not failing to think positively. You're not lacking willpower or moral fiber. You're simply experiencing the natural consequences of an energy-depleted conscious mind trying to compete with a fully powered unconscious system.

Introducing Awareness

So, if you can't outfight your unconscious mind, and positive thinking makes things worse, what's left? The answer starts with recognizing that your thoughts aren't the problem. Your *relationship* with your thoughts is the issue. Instead of trying to control what you think, you can learn to direct where you place your attention. This isn't about suppression or replacement. It's about creating space and redirecting your attention. Like training a puppy, you don't punish unwanted behavior; instead, you consistently redirect attention to what you want to reinforce.

This is what I mean by *awareness*. This word, which will arise throughout this book, is at the core of healing. When an unwanted thought arises, don't fight it or analyze it. Awareness creates the space you need to redirect that thought. Notice it for what it is and then direct your attention elsewhere. The thought might still be there, spinning in the background, but you're no longer feeding it energy.

This approach works because it recognizes the mechanical nature of these patterns. You're not trying to reason with robots or negotiate with automated programs. You're simply reallocating where you invest your mental energy. To fully grasp why awareness works where force fails, we need to understand the fundamental relationship between your unconscious and conscious brains, and accept both the curse and the gift of human consciousness.

Your Unconscious and Conscious Brains

There are several critical aspects to consider regarding the relationship between your unconscious and conscious brains.

The Gift of the Unconscious

Hunger, thirst, fatigue, fever, a racing heart, fullness of bowel and bladder, and high blood pressure are a few of the countless warning signals traveling through your body and nervous system. Such signals maintain a delicate balance, being intense enough to compel immediate responses to threats while also allowing you to react to safety cues, such as satisfaction after a good meal. Despite the painful nature of many of these signals, we could not have survived or evolved without them. This incredibly complex signaling happens without conscious effort. It is what keeps you alive.

The Curse of Cognitive Consciousness

With language came the ability to interpret and describe our internal sensations—what I call "cognitive consciousness." We assign meaning to the feelings generated by our neurophysiology. Since we're evolutionarily biased toward detecting threats, we continually produce unpleasant thoughts. Attempts to counter "bad" thoughts with "good" ones are futile—a mismatch of power that's not sustainable.

The Gift of Cognitive Consciousness

Despite these challenges, consciousness offers us a remarkable gift: the ability to choose. When we learn to access our neocortex and make deliberate decisions by consistently directing our attention to what we want, rather than to what we don't like, we can stimulate neuroplastic change in the direction of our choice. You have the capacity and ability to create any life you choose from this second on.

Ask yourself, "If I am spending so much time being anxious or upset, am I really alive? Or am I just reliving my past?" It becomes rather tedious to play the same music over and over again. Life is today. This has been known since the beginning of time. The true gift of consciousness is the ability to choose where to direct your attention and energy, made accessible through awareness—your relationship with your thoughts.

Summary

The curse of consciousness lies not in our ability to think, but in our tendency to become trapped by thoughts we cannot escape. Unlike physical pain, which signals us to withdraw from danger, mental pain offers no such refuge. The source of distress resides within us, produced by the very system meant to protect us.

We've seen how our brains cannot distinguish between social rejection and physical injury, how RUTs carve deeper neural circuits with each attempt to suppress them, and how our survival-oriented nervous system memorizes every experience, pleasant or painful, without our conscious permission. This creates a maddening cycle: The more we fight our thoughts, the stronger they become.

Yet within this curse lies an extraordinary gift. Consciousness grants us something no other species possesses: the power to choose our response. When we stop trying to control our thoughts and instead learn to direct our attention deliberately, we access our highest cognitive abilities and unlock neuroplastic change.

The solution isn't to eliminate unwanted thoughts—it's to turn down the heat. By developing awareness and making conscious choices about where we focus our attention, we transform consciousness from a prison into a pathway to freedom. Your thoughts don't define you; your choices do.

The ironic effect is neither a character flaw nor a sign of mental weakness. Instead, it's a predictable consequence of human consciousness functioning in a world for which our brains weren't designed. You don't need to become a different person or fix something that's broken inside you. Instead, you need to learn to work with your brain's operating system rather than against it. You require tools that harness the immense power of your unconscious mind while empowering your conscious awareness to play a more strategic role.

In the next chapter, we will explore the physiology that drives RUTs and most dysfunctional behaviors. Understanding the complex nature of RUTs allows you to depersonalize it, learn strategies for redirecting attention, calm your nervous system, and create the internal conditions that allow for conscious choice once again.

CHAPTER 2

The Physiology of Feeling Unsafe

Our underlying physiological state shifts our perspective of the world.

—DR. STEPHEN PORGES, *The Polyvagal Theory*

While *anatomy* refers to your body's structures, *physiology* describes how your body functions to keep you alive. In other words, physiology is the living engine of health and disease. Your physiological state affects your mental experience and can also cause physical symptoms. Long-term threat physiology can damage tissues, harm organs and organ systems, and cause bony anatomical changes such as arthritis and osteoporosis. Both structures and functions are vital. Every action, balanced by an equal reaction, sustains life. The physiological state that keeps a body's engine running consistently is called *homeostasis*.

Consider a car. It operates smoothly when all systems are properly calibrated for optimal performance. Tuning and maintenance are crucial. You can fine-tune a well-maintained vehicle to enhance its performance, but if the body deteriorates from neglect, tuning will have limited impact. Also, consider the vehicle's quality. Are you driving a Ford Pinto that struggles to leave the dealership without breaking down, or a brand-new Volvo that performs reliably even in tough conditions?

We experience significant stress in today's world. Just the sheer volume of information we process daily is overwhelming. Our bodies, bathed in stress physiology, can be compared to a car traveling down the freeway in second gear. Eventually, the racing engine will break down. Calming yourself, especially in the face of adversity, is like shifting into a higher gear and slowing down the engine. We can travel at the same speed with less stress on the body. Proper care and maintenance is also essential. You might feel that you don't have the time or resources for this. "I can't afford a Volvo." Really? The price is commitment, training, and mastery through repetition. You can't afford not to. All interventions are less effective if you are not caring for yourself. Random medical interventions will not heal you. You must heal yourself.

Life Is Physiology and Coordinated Function

From single-celled bacteria to complex mammals, all life-forms depend on physiological functions. Human physiology represents the pinnacle of this complexity, as it requires multiple organ systems to work together in an intricate dance to sustain life. While anatomy examines the body's parts, physiology demonstrates how these components collaborate to keep you alive and healthy. The fact is, the car metaphor only goes so far because, as living organisms, humans are far more complex than any man-made machine.

Your body constantly strives to maintain balance—not too hot, not too cold, not too acidic. When you're cold, shivering generates warmth. When you're overheated, sweating provides cooling. Your lungs and kidneys work together to maintain proper blood pH levels, with each breath contributing to this delicate balance. The kidneys filter blood to ensure a correct water and mineral balance. Simultaneously, your body operates like a power plant, transforming food into energy through metabolism. This process breaks down nutrients in multiple stages to produce ATP, the special fuel powering all cellular activities. During exercise, muscles can seamlessly switch between different energy sources as needed. Your nervous system processes information at an astonishingly rapid speed. As soon as you learn to walk or ride a bicycle, you can automatically do either without conscious thought about each movement. Your body also possesses extraordinary healing capabilities. When injured, specialized cells quickly mobilize to close wounds and combat germs. During illness, your immune system functions like an army defending against invaders.

Whether sleeping or awake, all these systems work together like a perfectly coordinated orchestra, each playing its essential part to maintain your health and vitality in an ongoing symphony of survival. Life is function. Illness is dysfunction.

Physiology Precedes and Drives Thoughts

Emotions are felt in the body and reflect one's physiological state. Our behavior depends on how we feel, rather than how we think. Research shows that the body reacts to threats before the mind initiates cognitive processes, and the emotional system performs its role before we even realize we are in danger.

We have known this since 1884, when American psychologist and philosopher William James (1842–1902) and University of Copenhagen physician and psychologist Carl Lange (1834–1900) independently proposed that physiological changes precede emotions, which equate to our subjective experience of these physiological changes and are felt as feelings. In his seminal 1884 paper in the prestigious journal *Mind: A Quarterly Review of Psychology and Philosophy*, James famously explained: "We feel sorry because we cry, angry because we strike, afraid because we tremble, and not that we cry, strike, or tremble because we are sorry, angry, or fearful, as the case may be." In other words, emotions are our interpretation of physical sensations. Lange published a similar theory in 1885, in his work "The Mechanism of the Emotions." While Lange emphasized physiology, whereas James focused on sensations, it is remarkable that their insights were so similar. The theory became known as "the James-Lange Theory of Emotion."[1]

Modern neuroscience has proven them right. Joseph LeDoux is a prominent neuroscientist and professor at New York University, widely recognized as one of the world's leading experts on the neuroscience of emotion, particularly fear and anxiety. He found that the body reacts to threats before the mind begins its cognitive processes, with the emotional system doing its job "before we know we are in danger."[2] Studies show that all aspects of cognition are mediated, influenced, or even initiated by affect (emotional state). We act based on how we feel rather than on what we think. People make decisions up to ten seconds before they are consciously aware of them.

This is why trying to think your way out of a threat physiology reaction doesn't work. Your physiology is what's driving the car, not your thoughts, and that is why *you must calm the physiology first*. Once your nervous system is regulated, you can access higher brain functions such as awareness and conscious choice. Yet modern health care practitioners are commonly trained to treat symptoms, not the underlying physiology.

A Hornet's Nest

A hornet's nest is an apt metaphor for the way threat physiology drives thoughts. Let's say the nest represents your brain, and the hornets symbolize your thoughts. The inhabitants mind their own business, working together to build a home, gather food, keep watch for danger, and reproduce. Then, someone or something comes along and starts poking at the hive. Naturally, they sense danger and use the weapons at their disposal to fend off the threat. Swarms of hornets attack the predator to inflict pain, and they do.

The prevailing medical model focuses more on treating symptoms than addressing root causes. In mental health, RUTs are symptoms, and we often focus on engaging with the angry hornets and confronting them. We also attempt to calm them down. Meanwhile, the nest continues to be shaken. Additionally, consider that the nest (the brain) contains inflammatory cells known as microglia that heighten its sensitivity. How do you think this will work? It doesn't, yet we persist in pursuing this strategy despite growing evidence that it is ineffective.

The obvious answer is to stop shaking the nest. Your thoughts also need to be addressed, but this must be done in conjunction with calming your nervous system.

Defining Pain

There are many different types of pain. For example, your experience of pain will differ when looking too long at the sun, listening to loud music, spilling hot coffee on your lap, having your best friend betray you, contemplating your mortality, and coping with the loss of a close friend or relative. What does the word *pain* mean? There are five basic types of pain, although these can also be categorized in other ways.

Chronic physical pain, as defined by the International Association for the Study of Pain (IASP), is pain that persists beyond a normal healing time (typically three to six months) and serves no protective biological function.[3] It often involves sensitized nervous system circuits that continue to send danger signals despite the absence of ongoing tissue damage. The Apkarian Lab in Chicago, directed by Dr. A. V. Apkarian, is a leading neuroscience research center with a major focus on chronic pain. In this lab, in 2014, Dr. Ali Mansour formulated a new definition based on brain imaging: "Chronic pain is a persistence of the memory of pain and/or the inability to extinguish the memory of pain evoked by an initial inciting injury."[4] In the previous chapter, we discussed how pain is permanently encoded in the brain, and it is also a physiological state.

There are small structures within each cell called mitochondria. They serve many functions and are best known for being the energy factories of the cell. A set of biochemical reactions produces a molecule called adenosine triphosphate (ATP). When one phosphorus atom is cleaved from the ATP, it becomes adenosine diphosphate (ADP), and energy is released. Without an energy generator, life would not be possible. Under stress, the mitochondria fragment and break down, releasing excessive ATP that leaks outside the cell and triggers a highly inflammatory response. The mitochondria break down in three steps and regenerate in a corresponding three-step process. However, when stress is sustained, the regeneration process is blocked, and inflammation persists.

Dr. Robert Naviaux is an esteemed physician, geneticist, and mitochondria expert who has spent a lifetime studying mitochondria.[5] He has linked twenty-six chronic mental and physical diseases to this inability of the mitochondria to complete the healing cycle and regenerate. To heal, this state must be addressed and reversed. This is why treatments that are effective for acute conditions have limited value for chronic conditions such as RUTs.

So, chronic mental and physical pain have a common source, and addressing threat physiology is critical to every aspect of your health. You can break the pain cycle by learning how to provide yourself with cues of safety. Dr. Naviaux is also conducting pioneering work on developing a drug targeted at restoring mitochondrial function.[6]

Emotional/psychological pain refers to the intense and unpleasant feelings that arise from psychological distress, loss, or trauma. Pain is perceived and interpreted by multiple regions of the brain. These feelings activate similar brain regions as physical pain does, leading to genuine suffering without any involvement of physical tissue. There are two components to pain: The affective or emotional component is what you feel about the pain, and the sensory component is where it is physically located. The main overlap between the two is the emotional unpleasantness.

Social pain is the distressing experience of perceived rejection, exclusion, or disconnection from others, processed by the brain's pain networks as an evolutionary mechanism designed to maintain social bonds that are essential for survival. Dr. Naomi Eisenberger, whose neuroimaging study of social exclusion was mentioned in chapter 1, has been a leader in elucidating emotional and social pain.

Existential pain is profound suffering that arises from confronting fundamental aspects of human existence, such as meaninglessness, mortality, isolation, or freedom, which threaten one's sense of purpose and coherent worldview. Dr. Ernest Becker highlighted this issue in his famous book *Denial of Death*. He hypothesized that existential pain was the driving force behind many human behaviors.[7]

Nociceptive pain (physical/acute), as defined by IASP, is a protective sensory experience triggered by actual or potential tissue damage. It involves specialized nerve receptors (nociceptors) that send danger signals to the brain for immediate protective action. What is less understood is that this process is fundamental to our physical evolution. This system automatically guides individuals to act in ways that prevent pain and injury. You experience pain only when the limits of the respective tissue are exceeded. If you relied solely on the sensation of pain, you would be in constant discomfort and would struggle to function.

Pain: The Gift That Nobody Wants

Let's take a closer look at what life is like without a protective nociceptive pain system. Dr. Paul Brand's autobiographical story, presented in his book *Pain: The Gift That Nobody Wants*, illustrates the necessity of having a protective pain system and the consequences of lacking one.[8] Dr. Brand was a renowned hand surgeon best known for discovering that a lack of protective sensation caused the skin breakdown and limb deformities common in leprosy.

He gained this insight from his experience while living in India as a child and then training in orthopedic hand surgery. He took an interest in leprosy and carefully documented the patterns of deformity and the outcomes of his procedures. Before his work, it was commonly believed that the leprosy organism directly caused the deformities. (By the way, I knew him personally, and he was one of the kindest and most inspiring people I have ever known.)

His story highlights issues associated with the lack of a protective physical pain system. Later, we will discuss how many problems arise from humans missing a means to shield themselves from mental pain, and how this leads to a dreadful, vicious cycle.

In the first chapter of his book, Dr. Brand recounts the story of his missionary family moving to a remote area of India, where no one had ventured due to a deadly type of malaria. Unfortunately, his father succumbed to it soon after they arrived. Nevertheless, his mother dedicated the rest of her life to serving the medical needs of the people living in this incredibly isolated area. He later spent the initial years of his surgical practice in India, treating patients with leprosy, many of whom developed severe, grotesque deformities of their arms and legs. He performed corrective surgeries and kept meticulous records of his methods for both learning and teaching.

Leprosy and Diabetes

Since the dawn of time, lepers have been treated as outcasts, with their limb and facial deformities considered nothing short of hideous. Following the discovery that leprosy bacteria caused these issues, their treatment did not improve significantly; however, it became at least understood that this was not due to some evil humor or demon possession. Doctors believed that the bacterium directly attacked the tissues, resulting in disfigurement.

Dr. Brand discovered that the deformities were not directly caused by the leprosy bacteria but instead resulted from the bacteria damaging sensory nerves, leading to a loss of protective sensation. The pain system sends signals to the brain, which interprets them as indications of danger whenever the limits of a structure or tissue are challenged in ways that could result in damage. For example, if a morsel of food falls into the cooking fire, a person with leprosy would reach right into the coals to retrieve it. If there were an injury to an ankle, instead of resting to allow it to heal, a person with no pain sensation would continue walking on it like normal. However, the walking would eventually lead to the joint's disintegration.

When Dr. Brand returned to the United States from India in the 1960s, he started noticing similarities between the foot and leg breakdowns of his diabetic patients and his observations of leprosy. There were poorly healing skin ulcers, infections that did not heal easily, and severely deteriorating joints. Doctors believed that high blood sugar levels caused the problem. Dr. Brand quickly realized that it was the same issue that affected lepers: The sensory nerves were damaged, and they were losing their protective sensation. His groundbreaking work led to more aggressive blood sugar control, protective footwear, healing casts, and patient education to help patients learn how to protect themselves. He made a significant difference in many lives.

Congenital Indifference to Pain

Dr. Brand also described the problems that occur when people are born without a functioning pain system, a rare condition called congenital indifference to pain.[9] These individuals cannot program their brains to recognize what might be dangerous or safe. Their lifespans usually only last about ten to fifteen years because they often die early from repeated infections.

Dr. Brand received, as part of his work and research, a large government grant to develop a device that would warn people with impaired protective sensation of danger. He created a tight-fitting body sensor suit that would send unpleasant warning signals to the brain in the event of potential tissue damage. For instance, if a person were using a wrench to tighten a bolt and applying too much force, they would receive an unpleasant electrical jolt. The problem was that people didn't want to be bothered and would remove the glove, which led to them damaging their joints. After several attempts, everyone eventually gave up.

There has never been a solution for someone without a protective pain system. The issue is that this system is incredibly complex and operates in a delicate balance. Furthermore, the final perception of pain depends on the state of your central nervous system and your previous experiences. For instance, one night of poor sleep can significantly increase your pain the next day.[10] Consistently lacking sleep can cause chronic low back pain.[11] Arguing with your spouse instantly heightens your pain. Running into a bully at school might cause your stomach to churn. This list goes on and on. Why is this? Pain is only pain because your brain interprets it as such. Acute nociceptive pain is a gift that helps you navigate this planet safely.

Narcissism: Faulty Social Pain Receptors

Lack of mental pain receptors is a key characteristic of narcissists. Just as leprosy and diabetic neuropathy destroy the protective pain signals that prevent physical self-harm, narcissism could be seen as a condition that damages the social pain receptors that normally regulate social behavior.[12]

In healthy people, emotions like empathy, guilt, and social anxiety act as essential warning signals, similar to physical pain. When we hurt someone, we usually feel empathetic distress (sharing their pain), guilt or remorse (internal warning about our actions), and social anxiety (fear of damaging relationships). These uncomfortable feelings serve as protective mechanisms, encouraging us to stop harmful actions, apologize, and mend relationships.

Narcissists seem to have impaired access to these social pain receptors. Without empathy's warning signals, they can't sense when they're hurting others. Without the protective sting of guilt, they lack the internal drive to change. Without social anxiety's cautionary signals, they miss signs of relational danger.

Like a diabetic who keeps walking on an ulcerated foot because they can't feel the damage, narcissists continue destructive behaviors in relationships because they're disconnected from the emotional feedback that would normally stop them. This creates a repeating pattern of harmful actions, leading to ongoing relationship damage, eventual "amputation" of relationships, and collateral damage to family, friends, and colleagues.

The analogy also suggests why external intervention is often necessary. Just as diabetics must visually inspect their feet daily, narcissists need external feedback systems to recognize relational damage they cannot feel.

Now that we understand the five types of pain, and why protective systems matter, let's examine how your body's complex systems produce these experiences. Let's take a closer look at the nature of safety and threat physiology.

Gathering and Analyzing Data to Sustain Life

Every life-form sustains itself by gathering information from its environment through various sensors, analyzing it, and responding in ways that ensure survival. Continuous feedback loops enable precise adjustments of each organ system in the context of the whole body. The three main components of the physiological system are input (gathering data), analysis (the nervous system), and output (survival responses).

Exteroception

Your environment provides input known as exteroception. Your body has many specialized sensory receptors that detect sight, smell, touch, sound, taste, pain, pressure, vibration, position, and other sensations, and accurately gathering and interpreting all of this information is vital.[13] When the physical limits of a specific organ, such as your kidney, bladder, or bowel, are threatened or exceeded, your body sends signals that cause unpleasant sensations, prompting you to take action to address the threat. For example, you tolerate only a certain level of music volume and refrain from eating rotten food. We have evolved to stay safe by avoiding discomforts that protect us and each of our organs. This set of responses is called the nociceptive system.

Unwanted thoughts also act as exteroceptive input, even though they originate and are shaped in the brain. They are interpreted and converted into physiological signals. However, there is no automatic nociceptive withdrawal reaction like there is with physical pain. This issue explains why mental pain has such a strong impact on health and well-being.

Interoception

The summation of all sensory input to your body is called interoception. It is a complex system that allows you to feel your body's internal states.[14] This is how your brain monitors your body to maintain its stable physiological condition, or homeostasis. As mentioned earlier, there is a constant and delicate interaction between cells and the organ systems within the whole body. This dynamic process is continuously monitored and adjusted every millisecond. Typically, your body responds quickly with uncomfortable sensations—such as hunger, thirst, a full bowel or bladder, nausea, fever, or shortness of breath—to prompt adjustments in behavior and restore the body's equilibrium. When your needs are not met adequately, your brain sends out danger signals. Once you have met those needs, you feel safe and content.

There is a dramatic difference in your body's neurochemical makeup when you feel safe compared with when you sense danger. In safety physiology, you experience a deep sense of relaxation, contentment, and well-being. So, why don't we exist in this state most of the time? Creating a sense of safety is complicated for humans, as our language and consciousness, which are also linked to our interoceptive state, alter it.

Serotonin and dopamine are two neurotransmitters in the brain that counteract each other. Serotonin is calming and regulates mood, sleep, cognition, and other physiological processes. Dopamine is activating. It acts as a psychological accelerator, energizing and motivating approach and reward-seeking behavior—including anger. It is also central to pleasure, reinforcement, and addictions. The dynamic interaction between serotonin and dopamine is critical in stabilizing mood versus seeking rewards.

Anxiety is the term humans use to describe interoceptive sensations when they perceive real or perceived danger. It is merely a descriptive word, not a psychological diagnosis. It evolved to become extremely unpleasant in order to motivate flight or avoidant action for survival. When the threat passes, the body returns to a normal state.

But what happens if you can't escape the danger? Many danger signals, especially RUTs, are unsolvable with typical survival responses. In such cases, your body triggers a stronger response, which we call anger. The anger or fight response includes dopamine, which functions as both a neurotransmitter and a hormone. Since dopamine is a primary driver in motivation and reward, you will pursue your goal until you get it or are exhausted. It drives addiction, which involves other activating systems. So, anger is not only powerful but also addictive. In this state, your body feels like you have nothing to lose, and your physiology becomes activated, often out of proportion to a perceived threat. The term describing this somewhat unstable state is *dysregulated*.

It is important to depersonalize these reactions—we are all capable of them. They are meant to protect you. It might help to use different language. Instead of saying "I'm anxious," say, "I'm having an activated threat response." Instead of saying "I'm angry," say "I am having a hyperactivated threat reaction."

The Autonomic Nervous System: Your Body's Balance Mechanism

The autonomic nervous system (ANS) plays a crucial role in the stress response and is located in the brainstem, hypothalamus, and upper spinal cord. The ANS controls internal organs and maintains a delicate balance of neurochemicals. It includes the activating effects of the sympathetic nervous system (SNS) and the calming effects of the parasympathetic nervous system (PNS). ANS regulation is hierarchical, and according to the Polyvagal Theory, three adaptive circuits work in concert to maintain homeostasis (balance): (1) ventral vagal (social engagement), (2) SNS (mobilization), (3) dorsal vagus (immobilization). It responds to the body's perception of threat or safety. The term *autonomic* comes from the fact that it works automatically, well below conscious awareness. Part of its function is to create sensations that drive behavior. Hunger and thirst are examples.

For over forty years, Dr. Stephen Porges has studied and emphasized the role of the autonomic nervous system in regulating bodily functions. His perspective includes evolutionary biology, physiology, the immune system, anatomy, neuroscience, and metabolism (fuel consumption). He offers a framework for understanding the complex nature of sustaining life and helps scientists and clinicians better identify the factors that influence chronic illness and disease. Health is function, and illness is dysfunction. This view is in sharp contrast with traditional medicine, which is largely focused on structure.

As mentioned earlier, Dr. Porges, Dr. Carter, and I formed an informal study group in 2020. Our group has grown to over 500 members and includes clinicians from various health care disciplines. As our group heard about their work on peptides and the autonomic nervous system viewed through the Polyvagal Theory, the clinicians were stunned. Threat physiology explains most chronic mental and physical illnesses, and this concept was new to us. Dr. Porges coined *Polyvagal Theory* because there are two parts to the vagus nerve. One called the ventral vagus provides function above the diaphragm, and the dorsal vagus affects functions mainly below the diaphragm. The Dynamic Healing model emerged out of this collective body of work. It is discussed in greater detail in chapter 5 and referenced throughout this book.

He wished to emphasize that references to the ventral and dorsal vagal systems as acting "above" or "below the diaphragm" describe their predominant functional domains, not an exact anatomical boundary.[15]

The SNS prepares your body for action by increasing your heart rate, blood pressure, and breathing rate, while also directing blood flow to your muscles and boosting sensory awareness. Often called the "fight or flight" system, it also controls vital daily functions, such as regulating blood pressure and body temperature. In medicine, *sympathetic tone* is the term commonly used to refer to the SNS's constant baseline level of activity.

The SNS is distributed throughout your entire body. For example, a pair of sympathetic chains, which look like beads on a string, run the full length of both sides of the spinal column. Each bead contains neurons of the sympathetic nervous system.

The PNS promotes "rest and digest" or "feed and breed" functions by slowing the heart rate, increasing intestinal activity, enhancing digestion, and facilitating recovery. It is mainly mediated through the vagus nerve, which connects the brain to most major organs. When the PNS is dominant, you feel calm, socially connected, and restored.

Almost 80 percent of parasympathetic activity is mediated through the vagus nerve. The longest nerve in the body originates in the lowest part of the brainstem called the medulla oblongata and connects to every internal organ.[16] The ventral vagal complex integrates with cranial nerves V, VII, IX, X, and XI, coordinating facial expression, prosody, vocalization, and cardiac regulation—collectively forming the social engagement system that supports communication and physiological safety. The dorsal vagal pathway, under safe conditions, supports digestion and restoration; under extreme threat, it can trigger defensive immobilization or shutdown—a primitive survival response that conserves energy when active defense is impossible. The classification of affecting organs above or below the diaphragm is a functional rather than a strictly anatomical distinction.

A cranial nerve attaches directly to the central nervous system, while a peripheral nerve communicates through the spinal cord to the brain. There are twelve cranial nerves, and the vagus nerve is the tenth. The other eleven are involved in smell, taste, vision, eye movement, hearing and balance, swallowing, facial muscles, chewing muscles, pupil dilation and constriction, and regulation of the heart, lungs, voice, and digestive tract.

Neuroception is Dr. Porges's term for the unconscious neural process that interprets and integrates both exteroceptive (external environment) and interoceptive (internal bodily state) information to assess safety versus danger. It is automatic, pre-conscious, and detects cues of safety, danger, or life threat. This integration of internal and external cues automatically adjusts our autonomic state to favor connection, protection, or disconnection responses.[17]

Your response to every second of your day depends on the instant sum of all your inputs. Do you want to pick up a few items at the corner store? Think about the many variables involved in opening your front door, assessing your surroundings, dilating your pupils to adapt to the light, coordinating your muscles to walk, deciding how fast to breathe, and figuring out if your body temperature is high enough to sweat. There are two main opposing forces, the SNS and the PNS, even though many other variables come into play. Notably, both systems stay active and work in opposition to maintain homeostasis. The vagus nerve acts as a crucial brake on your sympathetic nervous system, helping to maintain this balance and prevent excessive stress responses.

Your Body's Threat (Stress) Response

Your body's response to the environment depends on the intensity and duration of your situational stresses. Your reactions are rapid and precise. There is no fixed point, which is why we use the term *dynamic healing*. The body automatically gravitates toward safety. There is a graded response to threats, which can be broken down into four levels:

1. **Protection:** Your body is guided to remain safe.
2. **Avoidance:** Any real or perceived threat is met with a swift response. This is the default mode, applying to all types of pain. The benefits of this approach are evident in cases of acute physical pain. However, when pain becomes chronic, its problems also become apparent. In response to emotional pain, you might try to sidestep problematic situations or suppress distressing memories. Socially, you might isolate yourself to avoid feelings of insecurity and anxiety. For existential pain, you might seek out various activities to serve as distractions from those thoughts.
3. **Symptoms and illnesses:** A prolonged threat creates chronic illness and symptoms but does not result in permanent structural damage. I define illnesses as reversible because once you spend more time in a safe physiological state, symptoms can resolve without leaving any structural damage.
4. **Diseases:** Diseases involve some form of structural damage resulting from sustained threat physiology. Usually, this damage is irreversible.

It is generally assumed that structural abnormalities are the cause of chronic disease. This is not correct. It is the opposite case. Prolonged and sustained exposure to threat physiology breaks down the body and has long been documented to cause essentially all chronic diseases. Most of them can be halted, and some of their effects can be reversed. However, there is often structural damage that is irreversible. Note dementia and Parkinson's disease are on the list of chronic diseases. Sustained inflammation destroys neurons in the brain, a structural consequence.

I was diagnosed with esophageal cancer at age fifty-five, but I was fortunate that it was discovered during a routine UGI endoscopy for reflux. They managed to resect it through the scope and then had me monitored every six months. Fifteen years later, I am cancer-free. However, stress took a toll on me and nearly cost me my life.

Threat: Sympathetic Activation

Fight, *flight*, *freeze*, *fawn*, and *faint* are common terms used to describe some physiological survival responses to perceived threats.

Stress hormones trigger reactions in every cell and organ. For example, blood flow increases to the muscles, sweat glands become activated, heart rate and breathing intensify, blood pressure rises, and blood is redirected away from internal organs such as the bowel and bladder. In the brain, blood flow shifts from the neocortex to the limbic survival system, making creative thinking less accessible. Stress hormones include adrenaline, noradrenaline, vasopressin, and dopamine. Cortisol prompts cells to release and utilize glucose (a key energy source) for defense. When levels stay high, the body uses up fuel, which impairs its ability to fight infection. This process is called *catabolism* (fuel consumption).

The brain contains approximately 80 billion neurons, each of which is associated with around 10,000 other neurons.[18] These cells do not physically connect and are separated by a space known as the synapse. Neurotransmitters are small molecules located at synapses that facilitate communication between neurons. Under threat, they are primarily excitatory (like glutamate). Consequently, your brain remains on high alert, requiring less stress to trigger and sustain the threat response. In the peripheral nervous system, nerve conduction

My Symptoms and Illnesses

During the worst part of my fifteen-year ordeal with chronic mental and physical pain, I experienced the following different symptoms and illnesses, all of which resolved more than twenty years ago. This is not a complete list. Even though all my cells were bathed in the same chemical environment, each part of my body responded differently, depending on its cell type and the function of the specific organ:

Musculoskeletal
Chest pain
Back/neck pain
Tension headaches
Migraine headaches

Neurological
Obsessive-compulsive disorder
PTSD
Anxiety/panic attacks
Severe depression
Tinnitus
Insomnia

Immune system
Migratory skin rashes
Severe burning in both feet
Chronic tendonitis
Unrelenting itching
Hyper-reactive autonomic nervous system
Heartburn/acid reflux
Palpitations

speed can increase by as much as 200 percent. For example, experiments have shown that people are more sensitive to pain when exposed to red light, which is perceived as a threat, than to relaxing blue light.[19]

The immune system is stimulated to produce various types of cells that defend against threats such as bacteria, viruses, and cancer cells. Cytokines are small proteins that serve as signaling molecules between cells. There are pro-inflammatory (Pro I) cytokines that activate or regulate the immune response. Perhaps you heard the term *cytokine storm* during the height of the COVID-19 pandemic. The virus was not the direct cause of death.

A Sample List of Chronic Diseases

Neurodegenerative disorders
Alzheimer's disease
Parkinson's disease

Cardiovascular issues
Coronary artery disease
Hypertension
POTS (postural orthostatic tachycardia syndrome)
Stroke

Metabolic problems
Adult-onset diabetes
Obesity

Autoimmune diseases
Crohn's disease
Ulcerative colitis
Multiple sclerosis
Ankylosing spondylitis
Scleroderma
Systemic lupus erythematosus
Rheumatoid arthritis

Cancer (Most are associated with sustained threat physiology.)

Osteoporosis

Although pro-inflammatory cytokines triggered inflammation throughout the body, there were more COVID-19 receptors in the lungs, and the excessive inflammatory response caused the production of enough fluid to impair or block breathing.

Chronic Stress: Baseline Sympathetic Activation

Being unable to rest is a serious problem that occurs when you repeatedly enter fight-or-flight mode without time to recover between acute episodes. Your heart can sustain life for decades because it rests and rejuvenates between each beat. However, it needs sufficient fuel during the short rest periods. If the heart beats rapidly for a sustained period, or if narrowed coronary vessels compromise blood flow, the heart muscle becomes damaged from a lack of oxygen.

Contemporary life creates an evolutionary mismatch that greatly challenges our nervous systems. From an evolutionary view, humans once experienced safety within social groups, where challenges mainly involved basic survival rather than ongoing psychological stress. Our nervous systems adapted to handle immediate physical threats, not the persistent, low-level stressors that are common today.

Today, we face an environment that our nervous systems weren't built to handle. Research shows that seemingly minor stressors, such as negative social media interactions, can trigger more physiological stress than traditional stressors, such as public speaking. This relentless stream of threatening inputs—or baseline sympathetic activation—helps explain why humans still suffer from so much chronic illness, despite our material comforts and medical advances.

What makes contemporary stress especially harmful is its cumulative effect. In today's world, chronic stress is often accepted as normal. People might not even realize they are stressed. Many take pride in being adrenaline junkies and think they thrive on the adrenaline rush. However, your body, like any machine, isn't built to handle this. Rest is just as important, if not more so, than exercise for maintaining physical health.

Parasympathetic Withdrawal

It is still widely believed that sympathetic activation is the primary response to stress, but research by Dr. Porges and others shows that parasympathetic withdrawal—specifically vagal withdrawal—is the initial and most common event in responding to everyday stressors. The vagus nerves constantly counterbalance the sympathetic tone, and this action is called the vagal brake. As the brake releases, there is more relative sympathetic activity, although you are not in fight-or-flight. This does not necessarily lead to an increased heart rate or other changes caused by stress hormones.

This mechanism is especially relevant for low-level stressors, such as rumination, negative self-talk, and unpleasant social media interactions, rather than for full fight-or-flight responses. When confronted with these stressors, the initial physiological change is a reduction in heart rate variability (HRV), indicating decreased vagal tone. HRV measures the variation between heartbeats using an active EKG. A steady, consistent spacing between beats shows greater sympathetic input, while irregular spacing reflects more parasympathetic tone. Your heartbeat is showing a more natural variation between beats, which is healthy. A more specific measurement looking at the impact of the vagus nerve on the heart is respiratory sinus arrhythmia (RSA), which indexes ventral vagal regulation. Greater vagal efficiency (VE)—the dynamic capacity of the ventral vagal system to modulate heart rate—reflects flexible physiological regulation rather than simple relaxation.

Sympathetic activation drives a more rapid heart rate with less variation. In this context, inconsistency is advantageous. This parasympathetic withdrawal then leads to a relative increase in sympathetic influence, impacting all organ systems, including the central nervous system.[20]

Imagine driving a car while exerting equal pressure with both feet, one on the brake and the other on the accelerator. Vagal withdrawal is similar to applying less pressure on the brake while maintaining steady pressure on the accelerator. You can carefully control your speed by adjusting the braking level.

The release of the vagal brake creates a distinct window of opportunity for RUTs. As we'll discuss in chapter 3, the dorsolateral prefrontal cortex (dlPFC), the highest region of the thinking brain, has increased metabolic activity. But it doesn't regulate itself well. Cognitive control is excessive, while higher functions such as judgment and abstract thinking are compromised. There is over-inhibition rather than disinhibition. As you spend much metabolic energy mentally fighting unpleasant thoughts, you'll physically fatigue, think less clearly, and have less cognitive filtering.[21] Hence, flurries of RUTs.

After experiencing vagal withdrawal, you will be more alert. As your perception of risk heightens, you press the accelerator. You accelerate, with the limits defined by the car (your body). There is still some vagal tone, but it is overshadowed by sympathetic input. You are entering a fight-or-flight mode. If you push the pedal to the floor, your body will break down relatively quickly if it stays there for too long. As you become angrier, the whole dlPFC is downregulated.

Parasympathetic Activation: Safety

Your physiology undergoes significant changes when you feel safe. Your neurochemical profile is markedly different from when you're in a threat state.

Relaxation hormones affect every cell and organ system. For instance, blood flow increases to the internal digestive organs, the bowel, and the bladder; heart rate, breathing, and blood pressure decrease; and blood flow shifts back to the neocortex (the thinking center) from the limbic system, which is responsible for survival and emotional responses. Your metabolism (fuel consumption) shifts to an anabolic state, where you store fuel instead of consuming it. Neurotransmitters shift from excitatory ones, such as glutamate, epinephrine, and dopamine, to inhibitory ones, including gamma-aminobutyric acid (GABA), acetylcholine, glycine, adenosine, and endorphins. Some play both roles depending on the context. The nervous system benefits from decreased nerve conduction speed, more stable neural networks, sharper neural signals from lower background noise, and neuroprotection. Anti-inflammatory safety cytokines form the foundation of health and wellness by actively terminating inflammatory responses, facilitating tissue repair, and modulating immune system balance.

Vagal Tone as an Indicator of Safety

A strong vagal tone serves as a biological indicator of safety. When vagal tone is high, the parasympathetic nervous system effectively manages the sympathetic response, fostering a state of calm alertness rather than hypervigilance or shutdown. This state is characterized by:

- healthy HRV, indicating a flexible and responsive autonomic nervous system
- enhanced ability to regulate emotions and regulate unhelpful impulses
- improved social engagement and connection with others
- better inhibitory control over the limbic system, reducing the impact of rumination
- increased blood flow to the prefrontal cortex, enhancing decision-making and creative problem-solving

A strong vagal tone also promotes what Dr. Porges refers to as "neuroception of safety"—the unconscious judgment that one's environment is safe.[22] This sense of safety is crucial for allowing the body to rest, digest, heal, and form social bonds, instead of staying in protection mode.

A strong vagal tone is a powerful healing force, and it can be achieved through practical methods.

Healing from chronic pain symptoms, including RUTs, happens when you're in a safe physiological state. There are many ways to support and strengthen vagal tone, and once you do, you can let your body handle the rest.

Social Connection and Isolation

Dr. Robert Dantzer is a professor of neuroimmunology in the Department of Symptom Research at the MD Anderson Cancer Center in Houston, Texas. He has authored over 800 research papers. One of his notable works is a comprehensive review of social influences on inflammation. He identified four factors that reduce inflammation: a sense of control, hope and optimism, positive affect or attitude, and social connection. Laboratory studies have shown that these factors can directly lower inflammatory markers.[23]

Dr. Sue Carter is a distinguished American biologist and behavioral neuroendocrinologist, renowned for her groundbreaking research on oxytocin and its effects on social bonding, monogamy, and human development.[24] She has dedicated her career to studying the closely related peptides oxytocin and vasopressin, along with sex hormones, and examining how females respond to treatment compared with males. Her pioneering work highlighted the impact of oxytocin on the entire body in both males and females. Oxytocin is a hormone and neurotransmitter that has long been understood to play a central role in childbirth, mother-infant bonding, breastfeeding, and causing uterine contractions. Dr. Carter, drawing from fifty years of research, has highlighted its role in creating meaningful relationships and positive social interactions. Oxytocin is central to the function of the ANS and is known as "the love hormone." It is also highly anti-inflammatory.

Humans survived and evolved through language and cooperation, supported by social bonds. This explains why we are naturally tribal beings. Social connection is not just a psychological preference; it's a biological necessity that significantly affects our physiological state. Social isolation or negative social interaction appears as a particularly damaging form of chronic stress. Few of us truly understand the extent of its effects.

Oxytocin, often called the "bonding hormone," plays an important role in this system. Released during positive social interactions, oxytocin encourages feelings of trust, empathy, and connection, while also reducing inflammation and stress hormone levels. It helps activate the parasympathetic nervous system, which improves vagal tone and creates a sense of safety in the body. When social connection is missing, oxytocin levels decrease, leading to more inflammation and stronger stress responses.[25]

The effects of social isolation deeply influence our biology, affecting how our DNA is expressed. Research has identified roughly twenty to thirty genes that control the production of monocytes, a type of white blood cell vital for fighting foreign substances like cancer cells, viruses, and bacteria. Social isolation causes an overactive form of monocytes, known as "warrior monocytes," which become overly aggressive and attack not only pathogens but also the body's own tissues. This leads to various disease states and symptoms, with anxiety being one example of this inflammatory response. Social isolation is known to significantly contribute to the formation of these cells, while chronic stress from other sources also contributes.[26]

The link between social pain and long-term mental and physical health issues has been clearly determined by research. According to a comprehensive 2018 Cigna survey, about 50 percent of Americans reported feeling socially isolated or lonely.[27] We live in a fragmented society. Surprisingly, the groups most impacted are Gen Z and millennials. The effect on mental and physical health is substantial. Social isolation has the same impact on mortality as smoking fifteen cigarettes a day and is even more risky than obesity. Another key 2024 cohort study involving around 13,600 adults over age fifty showed that they experienced higher rates of mortality, disability, and dementia when isolated.[28]

Social isolation creates a particularly vicious cycle. As isolation increases inflammation and threat responses, the resulting emotional states (such as anxiety, depression, and negative thoughts) make re-engaging socially even more difficult. Many people describe the feeling of loneliness as "crushing," accompanied by self-deprecating thoughts like "Why would anyone want to hang around with me?" or "I don't have anything interesting to say." Social isolation not only impacts our relationships but also directly fuels unwanted thoughts.

Summary

A key insight for understanding RUTs is recognizing the two-way connection between thoughts and physiological states. Thoughts do not just mirror physiology; they also affect it, forming a cycle that can either make your condition worse or better.

When parasympathetic tone decreases, the brain's ability to inhibit activity in the limbic system lessens. As a result, the frontal cortex, which usually helps to regulate emotional responses and suppress unwanted thoughts, becomes less effective. This makes managing ruminations harder, negative thoughts seem more convincing, and emotional reactions grow stronger. Then, rumination causes more parasympathetic withdrawal, creating a cycle that is hard to break. This explains why trying to "think your way out" of rumination often fails—the very act of grappling with these thoughts can further lower vagal tone, making the thoughts even more persistent.

Understanding this bidirectional relationship explains why effective interventions must focus on calming the physiology first, using techniques such as breathing, movement, or social engagement, rather than directly addressing thoughts. Restoring proper autonomic balance naturally improves the ability to handle challenging thoughts.

Perhaps the most widespread and dangerous threat is feeling trapped by our thoughts. We can't escape them, and it's intolerable. Suppressing unpleasant thoughts triggers the threat response even more than acknowledging those thoughts directly. This suppression decreases the size of the hippocampus, the brain's memory center, and increases cravings for opioids.

You cannot conquer the sensations caused by threat physiology, nor can you escape them. They are always active. Once the sympathetic nervous system is triggered, it must be balanced by the calming parasympathetic system. The balance between these two systems determines your ability to rest, recover, and heal. In other words, the more time you feel safe, the better.

In the coming chapters, our efforts will focus on developing skills to regulate physiology instead of trying to control it. Our baseline always involves some level of threat, with alertness being the minimum. How effectively can we generate "cues of safety"? Recognizing and acknowledging our threats—whether real, imagined, anticipated, or repressed—is the first step in dealing with them.

The most stressful things are those that make us feel trapped. RUTs fall into that category. Our repeated attempts to escape from them often lead to anger, which can cause harmful behaviors toward ourselves and others. In the next chapter, we will take a deeper dive into "our dark side"—or what I call the survival quartet of anxiety, anger, schadenfreude, and envy.

CHAPTER 3

The Survival Quartet: Anxiety, Envy, Anger, Schadenfreude

One does not become enlightened by imagining figures of light, but by making the darkness conscious.

—CARL JUNG, *Alchemical Studies*

The need to feel and be safe is a deep, driving force for all life. However, it is not, by any means, a given that you'll be safe. Life is competitive and living creatures are always on alert. For example, dolphins and whales sleep with one eye open. Many animals live in caves or burrows. Horses and giraffes can sleep standing up. Countless creatures communicate warning signals and form groups to defend themselves against predators. Humans share the same basic needs of sheltering and defending ourselves from external threats. One trait that sets us apart dramatically from other species is complex language, which extends our communication skills far beyond those of other species and enables cooperation that improves our odds of survival. However, an additional level of conceptual thinking creates perceived threats that we have not learned to process well.

Your body's alert system is like a personal brain scanner, and it cannot be turned off. Don't think that solving a given problem is going to decrease your anxiety for any length of time. Your mind will quickly find another target. When you don't feel safe, you'll experience the survival quartet, always beginning with anxiety. These core survival responses dominate human emotional experiences, all serving the same fundamental purpose of keeping you alive in a threatening world.

- **Anxiety** = "Threat might be coming" (hypervigilance for danger).
- **Envy** = "Need more resources to survive" (pain of having less than others).
- **Anger** = "Threat is here now" (fight response to eliminate danger).
- **Schadenfreude** = "Threat has been neutralized" (reward for competitor's downfall).

Each of these sensations is created by your physiological state. We have no cognitive control over these powerful reactions—none at all. They are not psychological constructs, nor moral categories; they are biological functions. Your powerful physiology drives behaviors more than conscious interpretation. Much of human cruelty and harmful behavior does not emerge from inherent evil but rather from individuals caught in cascading cycles of personalized survival responses.

Anxiety evolved to be deeply unpleasant. Words fail to convey the depth of discomfort, which you'll do nearly anything to avoid or escape. Anger is even more powerful and addictive, and it masks the feelings of fear. It has also evolved to be destructive, since it is a last-ditch survival reaction. Schadenfreude feels good.[1] When you watch someone else fail or suffer, your brain's pleasure circuits light up. It is a more intense reaction if the person is a competitor or someone you dislike. This is your body's reaction to winning; it indicates that you have increased your odds of survival. All of these sensations are disruptive to your peace of mind and create a sense of uneasiness about your identity and values. But your body is simply doing its job of protecting you.

Most bad behavior and RUTs stem from taking survival responses personally. Without awareness of alternative paths, we often suppress or repress these sensations quickly. However, suppressing disconcerting thoughts and emotions intensifies threat physiology, shrinks the memory center of the brain, increases opioid craving, and creates generalized chaos in both the body and the brain.[2] Suppression refers to a conscious action, whereas repression is automatic and below the level of your consciousness. Suppression, as a maladaptive control tactic, will come up frequently throughout the rest of this book.

A vital first step in calming your nervous system, as we will address further in chapter 7, is to separate your identity from these survival reactions. Anxiety, envy, anger, and schadenfreude are sensations that you have, not who you are.

Another critical step is to allow yourself to feel them deeply, even allow yourself to react. But when you're in a reaction, train yourself to take no verbal or physical action, except in proper self-defense. Use your skills to calm down as quickly as you can to avoid acting out in destructive ways. Not feeling them means you are suppressing them. You must feel where you are before you can change direction. There are many words to describe these physiological sensations, but I have grouped them in what I call the survival quartet.

Anxiety

Anxiety is a warning signal that we must learn to depersonalize. There are countless other labels for anxiety, but ultimately, it is just biology.

Here is a word progression that reflects how anxiety typically escalates with increasing duration and intensity: anxious, alert, nervous, fearful, angry, panicked, paranoid, terrorized. *Fear* is generally used to describe an acute reaction, while *anxiety* connotes a long-term state. Anxiety operates like an overprotective security system that never quite trusts that danger has passed. The amygdala, your brain's ancient alarm center, scans relentlessly for threats while flooding your system with stress hormones—cortisol for sustained vigilance and adrenaline for quick escapes.

Meanwhile, your prefrontal cortex, the rational thinking center, goes progressively offline under this chemical siege, leaving you trapped in worry loops without access to problem-solving abilities.[3] You feel under constant threat with multiple physiological responses. As described in chapter 2, inflammatory cytokines increase, elevated cortisol levels burn fuel, and stress hormones stimulate your organ systems. Additionally, GABA, your brain's natural calming neurotransmitter, becomes depleted, while serotonin (mood elevator) drops, lowering your sense of well-being. Lower dopamine makes things feel pointless and pleasureless.

What began as an adaptive "scan for danger" system becomes a prison of hypervigilance, where your nervous system remains locked in sympathetic overdrive, unable to access the parasympathetic rest state that would allow healing. The system designed to protect you becomes the threat itself, creating a chronic state of anticipatory dread that colors every experience.

But one of the most perverse aspects of being human is that successful thriving relationships require vulnerability and trust. These traits are the antithesis of feeling safe. In the wild, being physically vulnerable can cause death. Herds of deer push the weaker members to the periphery so that they will be the first ones picked off by a predator. Humans also tend to avoid putting themselves in dangerous situations. But since emotional or mental pain is processed similarly to physical pain, and we don't like pain in any form, we find it challenging to feel safe even in close relationships. It is a significant conundrum for humanity.

Every interaction with another person involves the risk of rejection or hurt. Even asking a stranger for directions entails a certain level of trust that they want to help you. It's nice when they are in a good mood and friendly, but what if they are having a bad day? Deeper relationships—such as being on a team, working on a project together, starting a new relationship, or living with someone—also carry this risk. Being rejected at some level in any interaction is not only common but often inevitable. As you become more trusting, you will reach a threshold of vulnerability with that other person, and one of you might pull back or reject the other person altogether. RUTs related to rejection, acceptance, and judgment can become intense and even intolerably painful.

The best way to handle anxiety is to address the root problem that causes it. However, RUTs are not directly solvable; they tend to become worse when you fight them. Meanwhile, anxiety isn't easily managed through rational efforts. If you can't control your anxiety, what can you do? One idea is to create some cognitive distance between you and the sensation of anxiety by visualizing a large thermometer on a wall that shows your stress hormone levels. Instead of thinking of the feeling as anxiety, refer to it as "elevated stress chemicals." As we will explore further in chapter 8, several activities decrease anxiety by activating the anti-inflammatory effects of the vagus nerve, the tenth cranial nerve. For example, each of the following simple actions stimulates a nerve near the vagus origin in the midbrain:

- Rubbing your forehead stimulates the fifth cranial nerve (trigeminal).
- Humming activates the seventh cranial nerve (facial).
- Listening to calming, soft music engages the eighth cranial nerve (auditory).
- Breathing exercises directly stimulate the vagus nerve.

Clinically, Polyvagal Theory reframes symptoms of trauma, anxiety, and depression as adaptive physiological states. Interventions that engage the social engagement system—prosodic voice, safe music, coregulation, and gentle breath—support ventral vagal activation and restore physiological safety.

Anxiety = Pain

During my long career as an orthopedic surgeon, I focused on identifying anatomical issues that required surgical correction, with little understanding of the role physiology played. About twenty years into my career, over a period of two weeks, I encountered four patients who changed my perspective entirely. I was just learning about the nature of anxiety and beginning to understand the complex nature of chronic pain. All of these patients were professional men between the ages of forty-five to sixty-five with severe leg pain caused by spinal issues that required surgery.

On a scale of 1 to 10, each patient rated their anxiety, depression, and irritability at an 8 or higher, alongside reports of poor sleep and major life stressors—such as sick children, job losses, and marital problems. None of them seemed anxious to me, yet I asked each of these patients the same question: "What if I could surgically eliminate your leg pain, but your anxiety continued to worsen over the next several decades?" Panicked, they replied, "That would not be okay. I couldn't live like this. Won't surgically eliminating this pain alleviate my anxiety?" My answer was no.

When I offered to teach them strategies to reduce their anxiety by calming and rerouting their nervous system, instead of directly addressing the leg pain, they felt this was more manageable than suffering from persistent anxiety. These patients chose structured rehab over surgery. Within a couple of months, as their anxiety decreased, their pain either disappeared or became manageable enough that surgery was unnecessary. "Neurons that fire together wire together" is a commonly used phrase that emerged from the work of Canadian psychologist Dr. Donald Hebb in 1949.[4] The realization that pain, anxiety, and anger circuits are so closely linked changed my view of medicine. I realized that chronic mental and physical pain are essentially the same thing. Anxiety *is* pain, and it's a strong driver of RUTs.

Anger

A threat—a perceived or real danger—creates a neurochemical inflammatory reaction, which we call anxiety. This triggers a need for control to escape the threat. When we can't escape or neutralize the threat, we feel even more trapped. This spikes the body's stress response, and now we are angry. Simply speaking, anger is turbocharged anxiety. Both anxiety and anger are unconscious, powerful, automatic threat responses that we can't control.

It is even more crucial to depersonalize anger, which I also call "hyperactivated threat physiology." It is not quite as simple as turbocharged anxiety; anger carries a different chemical composition involving dopamine (reward), endorphins (pain relief), testosterone (aggression), norepinephrine (excitation), and decreased serotonin (lowered mood). It acts as your last line of defense—your body shifts into a warrior state, which is intentionally destructive. How many problems get solved and how many relationships are improved when both parties are angry? None. How often is there collateral damage? Almost always.

Anger often starts with a situation followed by blame. Whether you are the blamer or being blamed, you feel victimized and become angry. One of the most common ways to stay angry is by being self-critical and perfectionistic. You blame yourself or the situation for not being perfect. Now, you see yourself as a victim of imperfection, leading to more frustration and anger. Since perfection doesn't exist, you are always somewhat frustrated. Dr. David Burns, a renowned Stanford psychiatry professor, brought cognitive-behavioral therapy into the public eye with his best-selling book *Feeling Good.* He stated that the difference between your idea of perfect and who you are today reflects your level of unhappiness. In medicine, and in many other fields, perfection is often seen as a virtue and a standard, but it can be harmful to mental health.

If you were raised in an angry, chaotic household, anger might feel like a normal default mode. Isn't this the way life is for everyone? You might not recognize your anger if it is unconsciously repressed. Everyone has anger and suppressing it intensifies our physiological response. The range of possible consequences includes RUTs, addictions, and harmful behaviors.

Learning to process anger is always the tipping point for healing from any chronic illness. You might temporarily improve your symptoms but not truly heal because you have not addressed the underlying triggers of your threat physiology. I have seen this countless times with my patients. Here is an exercise I've had my patients do. Begin by answering these questions:

- What person or circumstance is upsetting you? Be specific.
- Acknowledge that you are blaming that person or situation for making you angry.
- Write or speak out loud to yourself, "I blame _____ for making me upset."
- Understand that you are now in the role of a victim.
- Write or speak, "I am allowing myself to be a victim of _____."
- Ask yourself these two questions and differentiate clearly between them:

  1. "Am I truly being victimized?"
  2. "Is my anger based on a preconceived story lodged in my mind?"

If you have truly been victimized, it will be harder to process your anger. The more justified your complaint, the more difficult it will be to let go, and the longer it will fuel your chronic pain. In a more abusive relationship dynamic that makes you feel trapped, you might need the help of a mental health professional or some kind of intervention. However, in most situations, you can pause and recognize the many ways you might be playing the victim role and forfeiting any sense of agency. Even when you don't consciously feel like a victim, learn to recognize the signs. Anytime you feel frustrated or angry or sorry for yourself, you are playing the victim. With increased awareness, you might be surprised by how many ways you are playing this role.

During my years of surgical practice, I thought that anxiety, anger, depression, OCD, and bipolar disorder were strictly psychological issues. I often referred patients to pain psychologists. What I understand now is that these conditions are not just psychological problems; they are the result of prolonged physiological states in response to a threat. I wasn't aware that mental and physical pain share the same circuits in the brain and are essentially one and the same. I knew that people trapped in pain were understandably angry. I concentrated on reducing physical pain, which exposes people to more mental pain. It was unclear why people would still suffer after undergoing a successful spine surgery. As I put my patients through a systematic self-directed rehab program (supported by the concepts in my book *Back in Control*) the outcomes of surgery were more consistent.

Your Stressed Brain

The human brain uses 20 to 25 percent of the body's total energy, even though it accounts for only 2 percent of the body's weight. In comparison, chimpanzees use 8 to 10 percent of their energy for brain function, while dogs and cats consume only 4 to 6 percent, and elephants dedicate 2 to 3 percent. Only dolphins match our 20 percent energy use for neural activity.[5] When the brain is stressed, much of this energy is diverted from the brain to other areas of the body to prioritize survival. This high metabolic demand creates a vulnerability: The body is unable to maintain high-level thinking in the neocortex.

Your thinking brain shuts down in proportion to the amount of stress you are exposed to. A friend and colleague of mine, Dr. David R. Clawson, coined the term *sapiocortex* to refer to the highest-thinking functions of the brain. He is a physical medicine and rehabilitation physician who has been a core member of our informal scientific study group. He has a remarkable grasp of evolutionary biology and modern neuroscience research. Current terminology doesn't convey how the thinking centers go offline, shutting down in a sequence.

Understanding brain anatomy helps us to grasp how this process works. The cortex is the whole outer layer of the brain. The neocortex constitutes 90 percent of the cortex, and it evolved more recently. The frontal lobe is one of four lobes of the brain, and it's located in front. The prefrontal cortex (PFC) is the front part of the frontal lobe. When we refer to the frontal lobe shutting down, it is too general of a term. Under stress, functions of the brain are compromised in a reverse sequence, with the highest functions going first. *Sapiocortex* refers to a part of the PFC called the dorsolateral prefrontal cortex (dlPFC) and several tightly connected regions.

The PFC is in charge of executive functions such as thinking and problem-solving.[6] What we will now refer to as the sapiocortex is the most recently evolved part of the PFC, and is particularly vulnerable to stress inflammation. Functions that are affected are working memory, abstract thinking, and thoughtful regulation of attention, action, and emotion. Mental flexibility becomes more rigid, compromising complex planning and problem-solving. It is specifically the association cortex of the frontal lobe that integrates information from various sensory, motor, and emotional sources, enabling complex cognitive processes.

The next region to go offline is the ventromedial prefrontal cortex (vmPFC). This is important because it is the bridge between higher thinking and emotional regulation. You become progressively more reactive based on feelings and less responsive to reason. The next region of the prefrontal cortex that is affected is called the orbital prefrontal cortex (OFC). Social behavior, reward processing, and behavioral flexibility become impaired. Then, the limbic system, commonly known as the fear center, becomes dominant as the upper brain loses control of it.[7] Emotional reactivity spikes, you are threat-focused, and social interactions deteriorate. In the final survival mode, only the primitive brainstem is functional for basic life support.

This hierarchical shutdown follows evolutionary logic: Newer brain systems shut down first, allowing older, faster survival circuits to take control. The sapiocortex—our capacity for wisdom—is humanity's newest and most vulnerable neural achievement.

Anger: The Doorway to RUTs

However, the greater danger happens when rational thinking shuts down and beliefs are formed in the insula—the brain region that processes internal body sensations.[8] It is a region that is *not* part of the PFC; it is part of the lower limbic system. The insula plays a crucial role in rigid, illogical pattern formation through several interconnected mechanisms. It monitors your internal bodily signals and determines what deserves attention and its emotional significance. It processes both physical and mental pain and creates expectations about the future based on the past. It can get stuck in a predictive error loop expecting threat or pain, creating self-fulfilling prophecies. The insula has extensive connections to the PFC, and a dysregulated insula can hijack and overwhelm the PFC, making logical thinking difficult.

With the PFC bypassed, there is little capacity for flexible reasoning, and the insula creates embodied beliefs that seem like physical truths.

When people learn information under stress, they cannot filter it through their thinking brain and are likely to believe almost anything. These insula-based beliefs are concrete, are simple, and feel physically real. That's a core reason why you often cannot change a person's deeply ingrained beliefs through rational conversation. We all know how pointless it is to discuss opposing views on topics like religion, politics, race, and life outlooks. It's nearly impossible to examine them logically and effect change, even after the nervous system calms and higher thinking resumes.

This is why authoritarian figures throughout history have been able to take control of a populace by creating societal chaos—a lot of it. Many of them have instigated wars. At a minimum, there is always a group chosen to scapegoat and blame, which is the essence of anger. Almost any group will do, as long as its traits are recognizable. The angrier and more reactive the population becomes, the deeper the lies that can be told—and not only believed but also deeply embedded. On a societal level, the repeated threat activation of neural pathways is all the more destructive and deadly.

To step out of this cycle, you need to train yourself to become aware of your physiology. When you're upset, blood flow to your rational sapiocortex decreases significantly. As a result, you can't access your highest thinking brain, and any actions you take could have serious long-term effects. While in this state, you might not even realize it, which makes the problem worse. Anger blocks abstract thinking, reasoning, and awareness while it fuels racing thoughts and RUTs. So, how can you handle this situation? There is only one choice: disengage. What are your other choices? Why keep fighting battles you have no chance of winning? It might sound impossible to stop fighting, but it is much easier than fighting endless battles. Have you noticed that there is never a good ending to a prolonged argument? One person might prevail, but the relationship is damaged. Arguing in anger is much different than having a lively debate or discussion about the details of a problem.

Since you cannot control anger directly, the first step is to separate from your thoughts and regulate your body. You need to recognize that you are upset and admit that you're not thinking clearly. I have a helpful phrase: *No action in a reaction*. When you're angry, no matter how focused or clear-minded you feel, you're not. You are in reactive mode. So, just stop. Don't say or do anything—and if needed, leave the room. It is futile to try to fight your anger head-on. Anger is a powerful and addictive threat response, and no amount of rationalization or suppression will fix it. In the heat of the moment, it's what you *don't* do that makes all the difference.

Here is another helpful expression: *Flip the switch*. Simply choose not to stay in the victim role. Step outside of it and move forward. It's a deep, clear decision made in the moment, and it works remarkably well. At first, it might be hard to give up the victim role, which can feel familiar, and thus paradoxically safe, but staying there will only deepen your anger and prevent real healing. With practice, it becomes easier to flip the switch. You might have to flip the switch dozens of times a day, but eventually you'll be triggered less often and be in that victimized state for shorter periods. This is a strategy you can use for life.

Anger isn't going away, and you can't beat it. The key is not to fan the flames when it does erupt, but to separate from your RUTs and calm your physiology, which we will discuss further in chapters 7 and 8. Healing happens as you reactivate your higher-level thinking, on your own terms.

Anger is your last-line defense and protector. It will keep you safe if you use it wisely. But learn to discern between actual threats versus perceived ones—and stay mindful of the goal of any survival response: to return you to a state of safety and regeneration. When your brain is in this highly stressed state, both you and those around you feel unsafe.

Schadenfreude

Brain imaging studies reveal an uncomfortable truth about human nature. When we see others fail, we often feel a surge of pleasure. This isn't a moral flaw; it's part of our evolutionary wiring and an addictive trait. For our ancestors, when competing for food during harsh winters, watching others' misfortunes meant more resources for their families' survival. The same principle applies throughout the animal kingdom. Many species express relief when a rival falls. Our brains have a more complex concept of threat, and we have learned to see others' failures as opportunities. Today, that same pleasure circuitry activates when we watch horror movies, root for underdogs, or feel satisfaction when an annoying coworker or abusive boss gets fired.

When someone experiences misfortune, schadenfreude triggers a neurologically perverse but perfectly coordinated response. Reward circuits activate with dopamine flooding the ventral striatum containing the nucleus accumbens—the same pleasure centers stimulated by food, sex, or achievement.[9] Yet, we've done nothing but watch someone else's pain.

The neurological genius is chilling. While pleasure systems activate, empathy circuits systematically shut down. The temporoparietal junction, which normally helps us understand others' perspectives, goes quiet. The anterior cingulate cortex decreases its activity related to empathy. The medial prefrontal cortex, responsible for distinguishing the self from others, dampens its activity. This isn't a coincidence—it's an evolutionary design that allowed our ancestors to benefit from rivals' downfalls without suffering a psychological cost.

Endorphins surge through the system like natural opioids, producing genuine pleasure while oxytocin—the bonding neurochemical—drops. Unlike anxiety or anger, schadenfreude doesn't flood the body with cortisol or stress hormones. Instead, it provides a neurochemically "clean" high that can even cause involuntary smiling.[10]

This creates an incredibly addictive mix: dopamine rewards without stress impacts, pleasure without effort, and satisfaction without achievement. The autonomic nervous system shows mixed activation, with some arousal from the stimulation but mostly reward-driven responses that feel completely natural and justified—making schadenfreude arguably the most dangerous of the survival emotions.

Vicarious Aggression

Schadenfreude occurs with or without envy. Without envy, it is called "vicarious aggression." It's a distinct type of schadenfreude when we enjoy watching violence without feeling personal envy or comparison to the victims.[11] Unlike traditional schadenfreude, which comes from thoughts like "I wish I had what they have," vicarious aggression is based on "I wish I could act with such power and freedom."

When watching fictional pirates, gangsters, or antiheroes inflict suffering, we're experiencing the aggressors ourselves, not celebrating the downfall of victims. Our mirror neurons activate as we feel their dominance secondhand, fulfilling hidden aggressive urges in "safe" fictional settings. We find surrogate satisfaction in forbidden power—the ability to break social rules, control others, and act without moral limits. The same neural reward circuits activate as with other types of schadenfreude—dopamine floods the pleasure centers while empathy for the victims fades. However, the fictional distance lessens empathic concern, making the pleasure seem more acceptable.

As a form of entertainment, schadenfreude allows us to indulge in dominance fantasies and aggressive impulses without facing real-world consequences, offering neurochemical rewards for watching cruelty rather than causing it ourselves. The risk is that, over time, our brains might become conditioned to associate human suffering with entertainment, potentially weakening empathy through repeated exposure. If you're feeling trapped by RUTs, which can lead to feelings of helplessness, this form of entertainment might create a powerful illusion of escape.

Envy-Based Schadenfreude

There are common types of envy-based schadenfreude that are found in nearly every aspect of life, appearing in different forms. The level of envy predicts how strong your schadenfreude will be. Research shows a direct link between these experiences. The more pain you experience from envying someone (dACC activation), the more pleasure you'll get from their downfall (ventral striatum activation). It's the same area of the brain that activates during addiction. You might not feel intense pleasure when in extreme pain, but you'll find some relief.[12]

Like other living beings, we are competitive; we want others to envy us, and, of course, we envy others, too. Language elevates this tendency. When we can't have what we desire, we often make it seem like we possess it all, which is one reason modern social media disrupts our peace of mind. Envy is also a normal survival response because having more resources increases chances of survival. Accordingly, the pursuit of extreme wealth comes with many social pitfalls.

Envy is a trait that is deeply rooted in our brains. It activates the same neural pathways as physical pain, especially in the anterior cingulate cortex (ACC). When we see someone with advantages we desire but cannot

Pirates of the Caribbean

While in medical school, I visited Disneyland in 1980 with several classmates. One of my favorite rides was Pirates of the Caribbean. I enjoyed the music, art, and the overall excitement of it all. But at one point, I started to examine the pirate scenes more closely.

As we approached the large area containing a captured ship, we saw a terrified, bound woman preparing to walk the gangplank. Behind her, several pirates gleefully observed as they readied their next victim. The scene of the captured town in flames revealed a group of young, frightened women on a platform being auctioned off to the highest bidder. Three or four women were chased around the burning buildings in an attempt to escape their pirate pursuers (they have since updated the bride auction scenes). Several pirates lay drunk on the ground, disinterestedly watching the scene unfold. Another prisoner was trapped in a burning jail cell, trying to persuade a dog with the keys in its mouth to come closer.

We entered the main pirate lair, and there lay the drunken captain, lounging amid piles of scattered loot. Numerous personal items, including toys, were displayed among the treasure hoard. I sat in that boat, surrounded by families with young children, everyone laughing and pointing at scenes of mass murder, sexual slavery, torture, and theft.

What had I been celebrating all these years? Incidentally, as recorded in *History of Litchfield* (published in 1897), one of my ancestors, John Hanscom Earle, was captured along with the rest of the crew of an American vessel by Algerian pirates in 1799. They were enslaved under brutal conditions and few survived. In 1801, Thomas Jefferson eventually approved the ransom for John Earle's release, but he was incapacitated from manual labor for the rest of his life.

These were not swashbuckling adventures; they were acts of terrorism. Yet here I was, and here we all were, finding entertainment in recreations of the worst human suffering imaginable. Why? What was happening in our brains that turned historical agony into family fun?

have, our brain interprets this as a real threat to our own survival resources. Social comparison causes actual neurological pain—not just metaphorical discomfort, but real activation of pain-processing regions.

This explains the overwhelming power of envy. The brain perceives social disadvantage as negatively as physical injury, often more so. The pain of envy drives an urgent motivation either to acquire what others have or to reduce their advantage and thereby restore psychological balance.

Schadenfreude reduces pain by creating pleasure. More envy increases schadenfreude. Unfortunately, envy gradually erodes compassion, leading to less resistance to schadenfreude. As a person gains significant power, wealth, and prestige, envy often shifts into a protective form. The individual in power feels like others want what they have and unconsciously builds defenses against envy. Compassion and empathy continue to decline.[13] None of this is a moral failing; your brain is acting to help you survive, and these circuits don't simply turn off after you've accumulated a certain amount. Our brains are constantly looking for danger, and we compare ourselves with those who have more resources. Then we counteract the discomfort with downward comparison to feel better. This destructive cycle can develop into an entitlement mindset, which is a type of mental rigidity.

Let's take a look at some common forms of envy-based schadenfreude.

Cheering for the Underdog

Evolutionarily, witnessing a rival's downfall meant better chances of survival. In today's society, this concept applies to corporate competition, political rivalries, and personal jealousy. Social media has amplified public shaming, turning it into a collective experience that releases a surge of dopamine. Consider how we view sports, often cheering for the underdog. Why is there frequently growing hostility toward a sports team that keeps winning championships?

Enforcing Justice

When a powerful or corrupt person suffers, people often feel that a moral balance has been restored. Celebrating the correction of a perceived injustice is common, which explains why public scandals, cancel culture, and political downfalls attract so much attention. Here's a more mundane scenario: How do you feel when a car zooms past you well over the speed limit, and five miles later, they're pulled over? Chances are, you experience a frisson of satisfaction that the driver did not get away with it.

Coping Mechanism for Inequality

When people feel powerless within an unjust system, watching a high-status figure fail creates the illusion of justice. It doesn't actually improve conditions for people, but it offers a fleeting emotional release from the persistent feeling of helplessness that simmers and disrupts the body's nervous system. For example, what is your reaction when an influential pastor of a prominent church is arrested for embezzlement, or a billionaire's company stock goes down in the wake of publicized acts of political corruption? Or when the fictional Robin Hood steals from the rich and gives to the poor? I am personally familiar with over fifty cases in which an office manager or personal assistant embezzled large sums of money. Some of them considered it borrowing and intended to pay it back, and they felt they were taking from an entity or individual who could afford it.

Active Schadenfreude

There's nothing wrong with experiencing schadenfreude; in fact, it's essential to acknowledge it, feel it, and recognize that it serves a protective role, helping to alleviate pain. However, engaging in active schadenfreude is a serious problem and lies at the core of human evil and suffering. The answer isn't to suppress schadenfreude but to learn ways to reduce your threat response. There are many proactive and positive methods to ease your pain through actions, like practicing altruism and cultivating compassion. These methods are discussed in chapter 10.

Tall Poppy Syndrome

Suppose passive schadenfreude doesn't provide enough pain relief. Then, you might choose to inflict pain. I call this "active schadenfreude." This takes the form of tall poppy syndrome (TPS) and bullying. Both types of active schadenfreude involve enjoying other people's setbacks. The main difference is that TPS involves cutting down those you perceive to be of equal or higher status, while bullying targets those you see as weak. The actions and outcomes are similar.

TPS represents our collective and individual urge to resent, diminish, and attack those who dare to stand out from the crowd.[14] Like a gardener methodically cutting down the tallest flowers in a field, society often seeks to level those who have achieved significant success, wealth, or prominence. This troubling tendency has persisted across cultures and centuries. TPS is envy-based active schadenfreude.

Dr. Doug Garland practiced orthopedic surgery in Southern California for thirty-seven years and served as a staff member at a world-renowned rehabilitation center for thirty years. As a clinical professor of orthopedic surgery at the University of Southern California, he published more than 120 peer-reviewed scientific articles. He was my mentor during my second year of orthopedic residency at Rancho Los Amigos in Southern California. Together, we published a landmark paper on the surgical treatment of excess bone formation around the hips, knees, and shoulders in head-trauma patients.

A few years after I left, he was responsible for most of the wards at this large county rehabilitation hospital. He fostered a high level of organization and efficiency among the services and was doing an outstanding job. One day, he returned from vacation to find that the administration had moved his spacious office to a tiny, windowless room in the basement. It was an unpleasant moment. His supervisors felt the need to undermine him and control him more tightly. He stepped down shortly thereafter and moved into private practice. It was a significant change. Instead of being thanked and appreciated for his dedicated efforts to improve things, he was

Tall Poppies: The Ancient Roman Origin Story

The metaphor comes from a story recorded by several ancient historians, most notably Livy in his *History of Rome.* The most commonly cited version involves Lucius Tarquinius Superbus (Tarquin the Proud), the seventh and final king of Rome (reigned 535–509 BCE).[16]

According to the story, Tarquin's son, Sextus Tarquinius, successfully infiltrated and gained control of the rival city Gabii through a clever ruse—he pretended to be fleeing his father's cruelty and earned the trust of the Gabiians. Once in power, Sextus sent a secret messenger back to his father, asking for instructions on how to strengthen his hold on the city.

Tarquin, suspicious that the messenger might be a spy, or that the message could be intercepted, gave no verbal response. Instead, he led the messenger into his garden and walked silently among the flowers, using his staff to cut off the heads of the tallest poppies.

The confused messenger returned to Sextus and reported this strange, silent behavior. Sextus immediately understood his father's symbolic message: Eliminate the most prominent, influential, and powerful citizens of Gabii—the "tall poppies" of the community. By removing the natural leaders and those who might organize resistance, he could secure his control over a more compliant population.

unceremoniously demoted without justification. Drawing from this experience, he carefully researched the concept and wrote *Tall Poppy Syndrome: The Joy of Cutting Others Down.*[15]

TPS has become so common that it feels normal. Once you recognize it, you will see it everywhere. A common and especially damaging form of TPS is gossip. Why do we do it so often? We all participate. We often compete for status in different areas, and we gossip to boost ourselves in our own eyes and in the eyes of others. We do this both consciously and subconsciously. A deeper driver of gossip is the schadenfreude response, where cutting down others physiologically reduces our pain. Unwittingly, we are reinforcing a strong survival instinct that is both rewarding and effective. This can become a dangerous cycle of needing to put down others to feel better, both physically and mentally.

BULLYING

Bullying is similar to TPS, but it specifically involves actions directed at those perceived as weaker. Instead of vicarious aggression (passive schadenfreude), bullying is a direct behavior. It is widespread and appears in many forms, causing serious harm. Two major studies from Great Britain, following individuals for fifty years starting in middle school, examined its long-term effects.[17] The first notable finding was that about 40 percent of students reported being victims of bullying. The consequences were severe, including decreased career success, broken relationships, higher rates of depression, more medical issues, and a reduced lifespan compared with those who were not bullied.[18]

Researchers studied students who had been bullied and those who had bullied others to identify differences in their physiological makeup. They examined levels of C-reactive protein (CRP), which is a blood marker for inflammation.[19] CRP is commonly tested to detect hidden infections. Chronic elevation of these levels also indicates a stressed and overactive immune system.

The study showed that children who experienced bullying had significantly higher levels of CRP compared with the average. Facing bullying isn't a healthy way to enter the real world. Even more concerning is that the CRP levels in bullies were below the average. It appears that there is a social and physiological reward for having more power. The implications of this in adulthood are clear. Why would anyone want to give up power and control, especially when dealing with the pain of anxiety? What's the alternative?

What is even more insidious is that we feel less pain when we bully others, but bullying can also be turned inward. It manifests as the self-critical voice that almost all of us take seriously. Self-criticism is a mechanical function originating from the lower brain, and higher-level interventions will have no impact without first calming our threat physiology. This will be further discussed in chapter 8. Consider your efforts to banish your self-critical voice. You might as well try to drain the Pacific Ocean with a bucket.

Every individual has a strong need to be accepted by others, and in children especially this need makes them vulnerable to intense social pain, when pain circuits are being wired for a lifetime. Now consider the fact that this same need to be accepted is what feeds the need to reject others. This creates an endless cycle of bullying, with anxiety as the root cause.

It is impossible to measure the full impact of bullying on our society, where it is widespread in families, at schools, and in many professional cultures. The suffering encountered at such an early and innocent age is profound and widespread. There are too many stories of bullying on social media that end tragically, often with teen suicide, that we don't need to go into here. But I've also had many patients and acquaintances tell me about their experiences with bullying.

For instance, a middle-aged schoolteacher told me she was experiencing total body pain and was a broken woman, barely able to lift her head to look at me when she spoke. She had endured severe bullying throughout her middle and high school years and couldn't shake it off. I found this conversation incredibly disheartening.

The son of one of my colleagues was severely bullied starting at age seven. Despite efforts to stop it, nothing seemed to work. Finally, at age twenty-five, unable to endure the chronic anxiety caused by the experience, he gave up and killed himself. As devastated as his mother was when she shared his story with me, she felt he was finally at peace. It broke my heart to hear her say that about her only son.

Bullying doesn't stop after attending school. It often happens in the workplace, where a person is singled out, treated poorly, and excluded. One term for this is *mobbing*. In the medical training world, denigrating medical students and residents is so common that it has almost become normalized. The implication is, "If you can't take the heat, get out of the kitchen." Compassion is at the heart of clinical medicine, and research shows that students applying to medical school have a significantly higher level of compassion than the average person.[20] It plummets during the third year of medical school, when the stresses are still minimal compared with those typically encountered in residency and practice. The medical field is not an exception; this cutthroat culture is common in many fields that emphasize high achievement. A strong predictor of disability is having a demanding boss.

Envy

Here lies one of the most tragic ironies of human suffering: When you're in pain, you envy everyone who appears not to be suffering. This triggers a destructive cascade.

1. Original pain (physical, emotional, existential) activates threat systems.
2. Hypervigilance makes you acutely aware of others who seem better off.
3. Social comparison triggers envy, which creates additional pain in the dACC.
4. Social issues magnify existing pain.
5. Schadenfreude provides temporary relief.
6. Counteracting guilt and shame about schadenfreude creates RUTs.
7. The cycle intensifies as each layer of suffering breeds more comparison.

The more you hurt, the more everyone else's apparent well-being becomes a source of additional pain. Studies show that people experience negative emotions like envy regardless of the actual difference between themselves and others, meaning that even minor gaps feel huge when you're already suffering.[21]

When you can't get what you want, envy grows, which then makes the pain worse. Talk about working in reverse. Like a squid squirting black ink to vanish, the envy that spreads everywhere causes your higher thinking self to fade away. I remember during my darker years, I became obsessed with others' seemingly perfect lives, wonderful families, circles of friends, and endless adventures. I was constantly comparing myself with them. This was long before the era of social media, which has now intensified the feeling of missing out on life. I can't express how intense this envy was, especially since I was already in pain. It was unbearable. It was particularly overwhelming during the Thanksgiving and Christmas holidays. I recognized there was something off about this mindset, but I couldn't stop it. It was FOMO on rocket fuel.

I understood intellectually that material possessions and experiences couldn't buy peace of mind. I had watched celebrities and very wealthy people self-destruct. One day, when I was living in the resort town of Sun Valley, a middle-aged patient broke down in tears in my office because he had sold his start-up for more than $50 million and now didn't know what to do. To say the least, I was confused. Around that time, over the course of eighteen months, six men I knew, between the ages of forty-five and sixty, took their own lives. Each was wealthy, had a good family, and enjoyed hobbies, music, and sports. They were also very friendly and respected in the community. This was happening in my neighborhood. At the time, I didn't understand what drove them to self-destruct. Of course, I don't know all the life circumstances that drove them to despair, but knowing what I know now—that research shows a direct link between ruminations and suicide—I have reason to believe that they were feeling trapped by their own RUTs.

Envy motivates people to succeed. Dr. Garland points out that there is good envy that inspires you.[22] However, bad envy also drives you, and creates more RUTs. There seems to be no escape. Envy-fueled RUTs were the driving force behind my suicide attempt, which felt like the only way out of my mess.

Envy is a universal and fundamental survival response. It mainly stems from the desire to lessen pain and the belief that others are experiencing little to no discomfort. When you face ongoing mental or physical pain, it often feels like almost everyone else is happier and has more than you. Envy appears in different forms, such as jealousy, FOMO, hoarding, violence, and anger—especially when we can't get what we desire or think we need or deserve. Sadly, many things we envy are out of reach for us. Even after achieving a lot, these feelings don't simply disappear. We still want more, including fewer and less intense RUTs.

Many of us have RUTs driven by ongoing envy. You might say, "I accept my life the way it is, and I am happy." If that's the case, consider yourself very fortunate. However, convincing yourself that you don't feel envy or greed is a sure way to trigger RUTs. These are not character flaws but instincts your body relies on to stay alive. To heal, you must connect with your darker impulses that are protecting you. You cannot eliminate envy and greed, but there are ways to release yourself from their grip and move forward.

The Core Error: Taking Survival Physiology Personally

Taking your powerful survival reactions personally is the core error that leads to RUTs. Understandably, you do this because your physiology affects every cell in your body. So, you might tell yourself, "I'm a loser" or "I'm a bad person." Not so. It is your body doing its job of optimizing your chances of survival.[23]

The human mind, with language, is less than 200,000 years old. Considering that we descend from 4 billion years of evolution, and that *Homo sapiens* walked the earth long before we developed language, we can deduce that language played a minimal role in our survival.[24] What it did was enable us to cooperate and become dominant in the food chain. We don't need a conscious mind to stay alive. As we developed complex consciousness with language, we gave meaning to our physiology, and eventually, our thoughts became another driver of physiology independent of our environment.

We define ourselves by our conscious mind, but it is essential to distinguish it from our physiology, which is largely driven by unconscious survival reactions. The main cause of human psychological suffering comes from misidentifying temporary physiological states as our true identity and acting based on that confusion. Suppressing these physiological responses is even more harmful, and avoiding or fleeing from them is impossible. An important part of healing RUTs involves using these survival sensations as clues that your body is trying to protect you, observing them with awareness, and consciously choosing to move forward. I call this shifting from *reactive* to *creative* mode, which we'll explore further in chapter 6. Each layer of personalization reinforces the original survival response, creating endless cycles of suffering.

Common Examples of Personalizing Anxiety

"I'm an anxious person." (identity fusion)
"Something's wrong with me for worrying so much." (self-criticism)
"I should be able to control this." (perfectionist pressure)

Common Examples of Personalizing Anger

"I'm an angry person." (identity fusion)
"I shouldn't feel this way." (moral judgment)
"This means I have anger issues." (pathological labeling)

Common examples of personalizing schadenfreude
"I'm a bad person for feeling this." (moral condemnation)
"This means I'm cruel and heartless." (character assassination)
"Good people don't think these things." (identity threat)

People rarely personalize envy or admit to having it. It requires them to reveal to the world that they are weak and want more. Since it is considered morally wrong by many cultures and religions, why would you admit it to others? Instead, there is a tendency to label the envied person negatively and cut them down.

Richard H. Smith is a social psychologist who authored *The Joy of Pain.* He provides a chilling and clear account of the forces in Germany driving the genocide of the Jews. Adolf Hitler was insanely jealous of the Jews, who made up only 9 percent of the population but held 60 percent of higher-level positions in business, banking, the arts, and politics. Since he couldn't admit his envy, especially as a supreme leader, he demonized them. It justified his rampant persecution and fostered schadenfreude not only among the military but also within the general population. The term is *transmuted envy*. Hitler and his staff were irrationally gleeful after every report of a successful effort to eliminate Jews. It was all based on stories they fabricated and systematically disseminated through the media.

This is linked to schadenfreude. Schadenfreude is qualitatively different than anxiety, anger, or envy—though it is fueled by all three. We unconsciously gravitate to it because it works well to reduce pain. The problem is that it feels morally reprehensible, which is why it might be the most powerful generator of RUTs. You could spend a significant amount of time and mental energy convincing yourself that you are not that person or feeling guilty about experiencing these sensations. But fighting it only gives it more power. If you use schadenfreude as another way to identify and separate from your stress response, you can simply observe and passively enjoy it and then move on. This will both release you from negative self-judgment while lowering the chance of it transitioning into active schadenfreude, where the real problems arise.

Cultivating awareness of when you are feeling anxiety, envy, anger, or schadenfreude allows you to separate from them and soften their grip. These sensations will always be part of your survival physiology, but with increased awareness, they will fade in intensity. You will be less inclined to engage in gossip, TPS, bullying, and self-criticism.

Summary

Suppressing any of the survival reactions—envy, anxiety, anger, or schadenfreude—is a surefire way to energize RUTs. Schadenfreude is our default way to ease pain, and there are strong biological reasons for this. It is a normal survival response, so you should not suppress the feeling or take it personally. Let it help you identify your survival physiology and move on with your day. Observing it with awareness in a nonjudgmental manner lowers your reactivity and lessens its power. It is critical to not act on it and cause pain to others.

The same holds true for anxiety, anger, and envy. Threat physiology is fired up in these states, and suppressing them requires a lot of cognitive energy, which isn't sustainable. Most human "evil" stems from people overwhelmed by layers of personalized survival instincts, desperately trying to find relief through increasingly harmful means. As this internal conflict grows and mental energy diminishes, behaviors tend to become more destructive. Think about your self-critical voice—probably the most harmful form of internal bullying. What if, instead, you learned to be vulnerable, removing the need to constantly boost your ego to defend yourself? Building and maintaining your ego causes a lot of suffering. Softening your ego is crucial for overcoming these patterns, as we'll discuss further in chapter 9. The solution isn't moral judgment—it's a clear understanding of, and a skillful relationship with, our shared biological inheritance.

When you stop wrestling with these feelings and understand them, something remarkable happens. You regain your energy. You no longer need others to fail for you to feel okay. You become the kind of person others want to be around, instead of someone they avoid. Most importantly, you become part of the solution rather than part of the problem. The person who understands their survival quartet as biological information, rather than a moral failing, is much less likely to act cruelly toward others. The first step toward healing any problem is awareness.

The revolution isn't about controlling our biology—it's about understanding it so thoroughly that we're no longer enslaved by it. When we recognize that emotions are a physiological phenomenon, that the envy-pain-schadenfreude-bullying-TPS cycle is a predictable biological sequence, and that we can interrupt this cascade through skillful awareness rather than moral judgment, we free ourselves from the exhausting cycle of taking every survival response personally. This freedom not only reduces individual suffering but also minimizes the ripple effects of dysregulated, personalized survival responses that contribute significantly to the harm humans inflict on one another. It's not about becoming perfect—it's about becoming conscious. And consciousness, it turns out, is the most powerful medicine we have.

Part Two

Stuck in RUTs

CHAPTER 4

Brainwashed by Our Lives

You are not responsible for the programming you picked up in childhood. However, as an adult, you are one hundred percent responsible for fixing it.

—KEN KEYES JR., *Handbook to Higher Consciousness*

"I have never seen someone take so many lessons, and practice this much, and have so little success." These were the words of my golf teacher thirty years ago, as I was returning to the sport as an adult.

I started playing golf in my early teens, although sporadically, and I dreamed of becoming a golfer who could consistently shoot in the 70s. But with medical school, residency, and life, I never managed to focus and practice regularly. When I began practicing in Seattle in the 1990s, I decided that this was it. I had some control over my time, and I met Art, who had coached a few players who went on to play professional golf. I took lessons a couple of times a month, and I enjoyed going to the driving range to relax after work a few times a week, which helped me make progress. I was able to shoot in the mid-80s, but that was as good as it got. Art was used to coaching students to a high level within a year. His above comment to me was made three years into my new golf life.

The problem was that I had developed a deeply ingrained, rather terrible swing, and as a surgeon, I analyzed every shot to figure out what I had done wrong. Of course it was impossible to develop a consistently good swing. I can't tell you how many golf magazines, books, and videos I consumed. I couldn't create a reliable swing, and on the course, I would become frustrated and self-critical. I wasn't having much fun.

As you know from the previous chapter, in this state, blood flow to the thinking brain is limited, blocking any ability to think clearly or perform well. I had become a "virtuoso at bad golf." The exact process that creates excellence can also lead to entrenched mediocrity or even incompetence.

This is precisely what happens with chronic pain. We become "experts at suffering" through unconscious practice.

Your Life Begins Right Now

The rest of your life starts right this second, and the next second after that, and on and on indefinitely. Your brain never stops learning. But most of your thoughts and actions today are likely based on what you have learned in the past. In other words, instead of forging new paths of learning, you are reacting to your past programming.

Human language and consciousness complicate this. Depending on how you were raised, you also give specific meaning to words that are connected with unpleasant experiences, and you have now associated those words with danger. Or you have learned through experience that something in particular creates conflict and discomfort, which has programmed you to avoid it. As a child, you have only a few choices: run from it, avoid it, or suppress it.

We don't have the capacity to stand up for ourselves and create our reality until our mid- to late teens. We cannot fully access abstract thinking and higher-level concepts until our early to mid-twenties. By then, whatever our parents and surroundings have taught us about what is safe or dangerous is well embedded in our nervous system. We are the result of who everyone else thinks we should be. Making a move to rebel against the past is still reacting to the past, which is running the show. We must find a way to separate from it to move forward.

Learning what is safe and what is dangerous—in all aspects of life—is essential for staying alive. However, anytime you feel anxious or frustrated, something in the present is connected to an event in the past, and you are stuck there. You are not here. Are any of us really alive if we are not connecting to the moment we're in? If we are spending our lives reacting, when do we get to truly live?

Twice a week since I retired in 2019, I have held a group question-and-answer session with some of the participants in my virtual course, The DOC Journey. One gentleman in my group was perplexed: "I am seventy-two years old, and I still hear my father's abusive voice in my head." He felt inadequate, like he should have known better. But his father's voice was there because it had been embedded early into his physiology and reinforced over a lifetime. If you are trying to prove you are not your parent's voice, this indicates that it's still running the show, and it is being reinforced every time you react to it. If you don't become aware of how your past is playing out today, your entire life will continue to be reactive, and the patterns reinforced.

These are deeply embedded, permanent patterns. You are wasting your time trying to conquer them. You might as well do battle with your refrigerator. This is especially true for RUTs. Each situation and sensation you have encountered in the past is connected with a thought, a concept, and a behavior. This all sounds dismal, and it is, unless you understand how these circuits were initially formed. Your brain and body change by the millisecond to adapt to your immediate circumstances. The descriptive term is *neuroplasticity*.

The fact that these circuits are permanent might sound discouraging, but isn't it liberating to know that you can give up fighting them? From this moment on, you can create the brain and life of your choice. The key is to separate from and not react to the past, and repeatedly connect to the moment. These are skills that are outlined and explored throughout this book, especially in part 3. You both separate from and crowd out the noise of RUTs.

Neuroplasticity

Your brain is the most sophisticated computer ever created, and unlike any machine, it rewrites its code every moment of every day. This remarkable ability, known as neuroplasticity, means that your brain continuously adapts and changes in response to everything you experience. Structural changes are occurring every second. They include the growth of new nerve cells (neurons), shrinkage of neurons due to disuse, an increase or decrease in the number of connections per neuron, laying down or losing layers of insulation that affect the speed of conduction (myelin), and functioning areas of the brain quickly compensating for injured regions.[1] The crucial insight is that you have a choice in directing these changes toward healing or deeper into suffering.

With the advent of modern brain scans that can measure brain size and activity, we can document these changes, which occur quickly. A study has shown that certain parts of medical students' brains significantly enlarge within a few months of starting medical school. It has also been shown that the brains of patients with chronic pain shrink. Fortunately, they expand again with the successful resolution of the pain.

Why would your brain shrink in the presence of chronic pain? Essentially, your nervous system becomes stuck on repetitive thought and pain patterns that develop into obsessive circuits, resulting in less time spent on creative ones. The brain area that enjoys activities such as spending time with good friends, listening to music, engaging in art, and savoring wine gradually atrophies when less attention is devoted to them. There is a vast amount of neural activity tied to these enjoyable pastimes that does not occur in the presence of unrelenting pain. Another factor is that under stress, inflammatory brain cells called microglia destroy neurons and myelin, especially in the frontal lobe. Dementia is one problem connected to chronic stress physiology.[2]

The bottom line is that your brain is constantly in a dynamic state of change, depending on how much it is stimulated, or not. There is incredible upside potential if you keep it active and creative in a positive manner. The terrible dark side is that when your brain shrinks or atrophies, as happens when suffering from chronic pain, you are less able to pull yourself out of the hole. It is still a solvable problem, once we understand its nature and start learning and implementing strategies to reverse it. It is documented that the brain expands when you heal.[3]

Geniuses at Feeling Pain

One of the books I always have had my patients read is *The Talent Code* by Daniel Coyle. Coyle is an investigative writer who has done an excellent job examining the factors that contribute to genius. He defines genius as possessing an outstanding level of expertise in any field. He looked mainly at artists, athletes, and musicians. It has been increasingly observed that genius is rarely born, and there is a popular idea that it occurs after about 10,000 hours of repetition. However, according to Coyle, it requires a specific kind of repetition called "deep learning." The other two factors are "ignition" (obsessive repetitions) and "master coaching" (repeating the correct actions to embed repeatable brain circuits). We will revisit all three concepts in chapter 12.

Deep learning is a fundamental concept because it involves entering information into your brain in a way that allows you to retain it. We all know that simply reading or hearing new information results in little retention. To improve memory, consider using techniques such as visualization, verbally repeating new thoughts and ideas to yourself, writing them down, analyzing and challenging the concepts, and reinterpreting the material based on your perspective. According to Coyle, by using interactive techniques you find comfortable, you can boost your learning by 500 to 600 percent. Conversely, random repetitions reduce learning by 15 to 20 percent.[4]

In short, actively processing information is crucial for retention and integrating it into your nervous system. Master coaching maintains repetition within a focused range. Practice doesn't make perfect. Perfect practice creates excellence. The reason RUTs are so problematic is that we interact with them in many counterproductive ways, such as fighting or suppressing them. You don't need master coaching for pain impulses, which are repetitive by nature. Why don't we have repetitive *positive* thoughts? Because we don't fight them, and we have not learned to embrace play and joy, which is a skill we can acquire.

Jack Nicklaus, the greatest golfer of all time, was asked by a reporter about a bad shot that had cost him a major tournament win. He looked at the reporter and said, "What bad shot?" He was so focused on his good shots, he didn't spend time analyzing his bad ones. I was taken aback by this statement. My strategy after a round of golf was to replay every hole in my head and examine all my mistakes and what I could have done differently. How much time do you spend feeling regretful about the past and not living up to your mental construct of potential?

One of my mentors is a successful businessman who began his career with nothing. He is the most mentally disciplined person I know; he simply doesn't spend time wallowing in negativity, even when experiencing some monumental stresses and failures. I was talking to him a few years ago about some significant setbacks he had encountered in his business dealings. I was telling him how sorry I was that he had worked so hard to achieve some impressive accomplishments, only to watch them crumble. He looked at me and said, "What are you talking about? The only question to ask is, 'What is the opportunity?' Never waste a crisis." He was legendary in his field for his creativity. He focused his mind only on solutions and simply refused to spend time in a pit of pity. He also pointed out that the world is programmed largely by negativity; why not make a societal effort to program positivity? He also told me how fortunate he was to have been raised in a nurturing home where this outlook was the norm.

You might say that this is a form of positive thinking and a way of suppressing thoughts. For many years, I said the same. However, a positive attitude and vision differ from positive thinking. Positive thinking is about feeling sorry for yourself and trying to talk yourself out of it to feel better. It requires a lot of mental effort and is a hotbed for RUTs. A positive vision is moving forward focused on solutions, regardless of the obstacles and how you feel. You simply refuse to feel sorry for yourself, regardless of how dire the circumstance might be. Why? Well, how does it help you to wallow in your misery? Where is the end point? Adversity never stops coming at any of us. You don't have to minimize or enjoy the challenges; just keep moving on toward your vision.

Think of a running back rushing toward the goal line in football. Regardless of how many tacklers are hanging on to him, he is not going to quit moving forward. When he is taken down, he'll have other chances. Interestingly, many of my mentor's strategies arose from his high school football coach who challenged him to think big, and then going on to play Division I college football. His approach is a way of flipping the switch and moving on. It minimizes your interaction with these pain circuits and reduces negative deep learning through repeated interactions with them.

Both of these approaches of simply refusing to spend time in a negative space are similar to learning a new language. To learn French, you must focus on words, definitions, structure, and grammar, as well as practicing a lot. It requires long-term commitment and effort to become fluent. But the most effective method is to immerse yourself in a French-speaking country—where you must speak it, not just passively listen to it.

The language we are learning here is "an enjoyable life." Our default language is one of survival, doing what we can to make it through the day. It requires a concerted effort to become fluent in living life on your terms, and you'll make many mistakes along the way. You must stay focused on your vision.

One experiment that illustrates the power of reprogramming is the famous one by Ivan Pavlov, a Russian researcher. Pavlov demonstrated how the brain can be trained, through repetition, to have specific reactions in particular situations. Recent neuroscience now supports his findings. Pavlov held an experiment in which the sound of a bell accompanied every interaction a dog had with food. Eventually, just the sound of the bell would make the dog salivate, even in the absence of food to see or smell.

One of Pavlov's lesser-known experiments involved coupling the dog's interaction with food with the application of an electric shock to one of its legs. With repetition, the dog would eventually learn to seek the electric shock to obtain food and would no longer react to the shock with a pain response. However, this phenomenon was "paw dependent" in that if the same shock was applied to its other leg, the dog would scream with pain. This experiment shows that the brain can be reprogrammed to adapt to almost anything.[5]

Any person can stimulate neuroplastic changes and program a new set of circuits. It is the reason that I never assume a person cannot heal, no matter how long they have suffered or how many pain symptoms they have. Over the course of my long career, I have seen many patients in dismal circumstances with no hope of transcending their pain. I can never tell who will or will not succeed, or how long it will take, but among those who have healed, I've noticed they share a common trait of engagement and persistence.

Take, for example, a woman I recently met, who suffered total body pain caused by reflex sympathetic dystrophy (RSD) for over thirty years. It is one of the worst pain syndromes imaginable, and I don't know how she got through it. Using her version of the concepts in this book, she became pain-free and has remained so for fifteen years. She is now a health coach who helps people out of chronic pain. Her term for her approach is "self-directed neuroplasticity."

Another gentleman finally broke free of his pain throughout his whole body after undergoing twenty-nine surgeries over the course of twenty years. Seven of them were on his lower back. Just before he read my book *Back in Control*, he had made a serious suicide attempt by overdosing on opioids. His rehab physician calmly kept asking him what he was so angry about. Despite years of adversity, he remained unaware of his anger. Over the following weeks, he began to address it and read *Back in Control*. When I saw him six months later, he was well on his way to healing. I continued to work with him for another year. He has been free of mental and physical pain for over ten years and reports that he has never felt better.

Another one of my patients had suffered primarily from mental pain for more than fifty years before healing and becoming pain-free about twelve years ago. The question her doctors never asked her was, "How is your life going?" If they had, they would have learned that her ex-husband and the father of her children committed suicide at age thirty, and the year her pain became intolerable, her forty-year-old son killed himself.

I mention these people's stories to show that, when it comes to healing, almost anything is possible. The common wisdom is that after eighteen months of chronic pain, there is nothing that can be done. This does not take into account the core healing concepts of safety physiology and neuroplasticity. Each person is unique, and there are different approaches to implementing these core concepts, but the key is to focus on mastering skills, not on the pain. Thanks to neuroplasticity, anything is possible if you stay focused on your vision.

Human Programming vs. Artificial Intelligence

You can think of your brain as the most advanced computer ever created, one that has been receiving input since birth. Both human brains and artificial intelligence (AI) process input, analyze data, and create outputs. However, there is a key difference: Humans possess interoception (body sensations) and the capacity to assess and alter each other's moods and emotions.

AI processes electronic signals but cannot feel a sense of threat or safety, nor does it suffer from chronic illnesses. It can create art that elicits emotions, altering physiology in humans, but another AI machine observing the same art will be unable to feel anything. Your body instantly responds to threatening sensory input, and thoughts follow within one to ten seconds. AI immediately responds to electronic data and can simulate a danger response, but it does not respond to feelings. There are only electrical impulses and no physiology to interpret. The brain simultaneously responds to multiple sources of input. But there is an important parallel between the human brain and AI—and herein lies the real problem with the human condition.

The effectiveness of AI depends on two core factors: the quality of the data input and the algorithm processing the data. For example, if you download the rules of chess into AI without clear strategies on how to utilize them, nothing of significance will happen. For AI to develop a mastery of chess, the data and the approaches need to be taught by chess masters. Only then can it analyze the approaches, mistakes, and good moves, and eventually outperform the master.

What if you input the wrong rules, or have it programmed by someone who knows the rules but can only see one or two moves ahead? There is little chance that the computer will gain enough experience to compete at a high level, let alone become a Grandmaster. The computer can improve on good moves but can also reinforce incompetence. In the business world, inputting inaccurate data into AI systems can be costly for an industry.

Now consider the quality of the data that has been downloaded into your brain, and what you continue to load in. What are the rules for processing it and making sound decisions? Once you start on the wrong trajectory, it will only worsen without better data and improved processing rules. Consider the extreme forms of poor input and coping skills from being raised in an abusive environment. All children need from their family is to feel safe and nurtured, and be educated and taught social skills. That's it. That is not what many of us get, however. So, the download in our brains from the beginning is "flawed data." We are not taught to process it; we are too busy surviving to feel safe, and we lack the skills to cultivate healthy relationships and nurture joy and creativity. Therefore, our processing system is riddled with incorrect data and analyzed by the wrong set of rules. The distorted outputs or behaviors can cause our life trajectory to spiral out of control.

Brainwashed by Our Lives

Years ago, the thought floated in my head about how our own lives brainwash us. I was becoming aware of how some of my unhealthy family patterns and traits were playing out in my life. These were patterns and traits that I was actively working on.

The following week, I encountered Jim. Jim was trying my patience. He was in his late thirties, muscular, surly, had injured his back at work, and wasn't happy about the way his case was going. Like many people stuck in the workers' compensation system, he was understandably frustrated and angry, having been immersed in it for over five years. I was viewed as part of it, despite my efforts to advocate for him. He was about six feet tall and 220 pounds of muscle. His fiancée was a petite redhead, hardly taller than five feet, who exuded an incredible, vivacious energy.

Jim needed a back operation for a pinched nerve that was causing pain in his right leg. He was his usual moody and uncooperative self. He hadn't followed up on anything we'd discussed regarding rehab and calming down his nervous system. His symptoms were compelling enough that I had signed him up for surgery, but he still wouldn't engage in any part of his healing process.

Finally, I gave up. "Look," I said. "I am going to cancel your surgery. I cannot help you if you don't want to participate in learning the tools I'm trying to give you to get better. It's just the way I work." I had a sense that Jim's resistance to stress management stemmed from his background experiences, so I also added, "We are all programmed by our past. For example, if you were raised in a family that was active in the Ku Klux Klan, what do you think your belief system would be?" His fiancée suddenly burst out laughing hysterically. It didn't seem that funny to me, particularly since I was so frustrated at that moment with Jim's lack of cooperation. I thought I'd picked a completely random example, but Jim looked me in the eye and said, "My father and grandfather were Grand Knights in the Klan." It was an awkward moment.

When I was a teenager, I became fascinated by stories of people who joined cults. These were not naive individuals; many came from good families and had college educations. Yet, despite the blatant abuse and manipulation, they found it nearly impossible to break free. They didn't even view their situation as a predicament. What puzzled me was how repetitive messages had effectively become their version of reality. They processed new information through a completely altered filter, and passionately defended their groups when outsiders pointed out apparent contradictions. Beliefs are easily confused with facts.

Being on constant alert works brilliantly for physical threats. For example, our ancestors who wanted to survive long enough to reproduce had to learn that certain plants were poisonous. We learn what's dangerous and what's safe, then we instinctively avoid danger and seek safety. But here's the problem: Our brains process mental and emotional pain through many of the same pathways as physical pain. When you were rebuked as a child, your nervous system registered that as a survival threat. When you were rejected or humiliated, your brain filed those experiences as danger situations to avoid.

If you grew up in a chaotic environment—with parents who fought constantly, struggled with addiction, or didn't know how to create emotional safety—your nervous system learned to perceive many more things as potentially dangerous. Sometimes they were unsafe, but often they were unpredictable. Your brain didn't make fine distinctions; it simply marked them as "proceed with extreme caution."

Family chaos can also be so rampant and persistent that it becomes your version of reality. You might think, "Isn't this the way everyone is?" During my first year of orthopedic residency, I admitted a woman with back pain and an anxiety disorder. I didn't know what that term meant and had to look it up in a medical textbook. At twenty-eight years old, I was unaware of the meaning of the word *anxiety*. I was perplexed that I had gone through my whole life not knowing this word.

Many years later, I attended a parents' workshop at my stepdaughter's boarding school. As I shared my childhood story of family chaos and listened to others tell theirs, it hit me: Anxiety was my baseline condition, the starting point and foundation for my life. It was all I knew. I had just kept pushing forward using my own blind coping strategies. I had already healed from over fifteen years of multiple physical symptoms, severe anxiety, major depression, and OCD. I knew many of the principles of healing, but I did not know about the driving force of stress physiology. Even though a lifetime of chaos seemed to be normal, the unrelenting threat physiology made me sick. This moment of insight was intense.

I've observed that some people fear change, or hesitate to try new ideas, regardless of how their lives are unfolding. They've made it this far using their existing strategies, which are familiar to them. From the perspective of their nervous system, why risk altering something that has kept them alive? Until your nervous system feels secure enough to consider trying something different, you're up against a lifetime of familiar programming, as well as millions of years of evolutionary programming that prioritizes survival over growth.

Human Dependency and Vulnerability

David Eagleman points out in his brilliant book *Livewired* that humans are uniquely dependent on their parents for physical survival compared with most mammals.[6] A baby is completely helpless and cannot survive on its own for many years. But our emotional and cognitive development takes even longer. We don't fully develop the capacity for abstract thinking, judgment, impulse control, emotional regulation, and other executive functions until our mid-twenties. This means our environment is programming us for decades, and we are uniquely at the mercy of our families' dysfunction.

Healing happens by stimulating neuroplastic changes in the sapiocortex, which is best accessed when you are calm. If you have seldom experienced safety in your life, you will find it difficult to access your sapiocortex, and it likely has not developed optimally. Fortunately, understanding how to create safety and stimulate neuroplastic changes can make up for your old programming, at any age. Grasping these concepts and applying them to your life requires persistence. It's not a temporary fix, but a healing framework that should last a lifetime.

Imagine the life of a feral cat that has lived on the streets for years. This cat's nervous system has been shaped by constant danger—every sound could be a predator, every human a threat. Its hypervigilance isn't a personality trait; it's a survival adaptation that has kept it alive. This programming runs deep: ingrained fast reflexes, muscle tension, breathing patterns, and sleep cycles. The cat's nervous system is programmed to assume a threat until proven otherwise.

Now, picture you bringing this cat into your safe home. Although it is no longer in danger, its nervous system remains unaware of that. It requires far less stimulation to trigger its stress response compared to a house cat raised in a safe environment. A sudden noise or quick movement might send the feral cat into a panic that wouldn't faze a secure cat.

Calming down this cat requires working at the nervous system level, sequentially helping it feel safe, then safer, and then even safer. This cannot be rushed. You might start by simply being present, consistently offering food, speaking softly, and moving slowly. It's likely this cat will always to be more sensitive than one raised in a safe environment. Its nervous system maintains a hypervigilance capacity, which could cause it to revert to old patterns under stress.

This describes humans raised in chaotic environments. Their responses aren't based on conscious thought but on nervous system programing that operates faster than awareness. Lasting change requires the creation of new safety experiences that gradually compete with old programing—slow work that necessitates patience, not analysis or willpower alone.

The Impact of Early Trauma

Dr. Vincent Felitti discovered something extraordinary while treating obesity at Kaiser Permanente. His program, which involved over 30,000 patients, achieved remarkable results: an average loss of sixty-two pounds through intensive therapy combined with fasting. But then something puzzling occurred: Successful patients began to experience severe distress, and some left the program.

When Felitti examined their histories, a troubling pattern emerged. Many had experienced childhood trauma, particularly sexual abuse, and obesity was not merely a result of overeating—it served as unconscious protection. As one patient revealed after connecting her 105-pound weight gain to a rape, "Overweight is overlooked, and that's the way I need to be."

Two key predictors of weight regain emerged: a history of childhood sexual abuse and being in a dysfunctional marriage. These findings laid the groundwork for the Adverse Childhood Experiences (ACE) Study.[7]

The landmark 1998 study by Dr. Felitti, Dr. Robert Anda, and colleagues examined the relationship between adverse childhood experiences and adult health outcomes at Kaiser Permanente in San Diego, California.[8] The study surveyed 13,494 adults, and 70.5 percent responded, with 9,508 completing the medical evaluations. Initially, the research started with seven ACEs, then expanded to ten:

1. psychological abuse
2. physical abuse
3. sexual abuse
4. violence against the mother
5. living with household members who were substance abusers
6. living with household members who were mentally ill or suicidal
7. living with household members who were ever imprisoned

THREE ADDED CATEGORIES:

1. emotional neglect
2. physical neglect
3. parental separation or divorce

The study demonstrated a link between the ACE score and difficulties in functioning later in life: The higher the score, the worse the adult problems. One of the most disturbing aspects of the study was that only about one-third of people had an ACE score of zero, while 26 percent had three or more.

In both the original seven-category assessment and the expanded ten-category version, four or more ACEs marked the critical threshold where significant increases in health risks were observed. This "dose-response" relationship indicates that the risk of adverse outcomes rises with each additional ACE, but there is a particularly notable jump at the four-point threshold. At over four ACEs, research consistently shows:

- 4- to 12-fold increases in alcoholism, drug abuse, depression, and suicide attempts

- 2- to 4-fold increases in smoking, poor self-rated health, a high number of sexual partners, and STDs
- 1.4- to 1.6-fold increases in physical inactivity and severe obesity
- increased risk of heart disease, cancer, chronic lung disease, and liver disease

More recent studies show essentially the same outcomes. One 2025 study showed that parents with high ACE scores created a home with high ACE scores.[9] Another study in 2024 looked at self-reported experiences in high school: 76.1 percent reported one or more ACEs, with 18.5 percent reporting four or more ACEs.[10] A large 2025 survey of 93,000 young adults born between 1999 and 2003 measured participants' outcomes at ages eighteen to twenty-two. The data showed that young people with high ACE scores have a higher chance of being charged with felonies, living in poverty, and having children in their teens, and are less likely to be educated.[11] Overall, our country isn't doing a competent job of parenting, and we are all paying the price.

There is substantial evidence suggesting that early experiences of abuse and neglect might be linked to an adulthood tendency to engage in repetitive negative thinking, such as worry and rumination. Rumination that reinforces negative concepts of self might be the mediator between childhood trauma and suicidal ideation. Research also indicates that traumas that have not been fully discussed and processed are associated with increased ruminations about traumatic events.[12] However, it's important to note that discussing trauma—in the form of talk therapy or otherwise—must be aligned with approaches to help you feel safe, rather than just reinforcing unpleasant circuits.

Just Be

What if you were raised in a household with attentive parents (or other caregivers), yet still experience more annoying, disruptive thoughts than you would like? Other influences come into play. Adults tend to be critical of others and feel the need to instill good values in their children, as well as teach them life skills to compete in the workforce. From a survival perspective, this makes complete sense. Children learn quickly and have open minds. They learn more quickly when they feel safe and their sapiocortex is online. Otherwise, new information will be learned without optimal filtering of information, potentially compromising long-term judgment, analytical and abstract thinking, and other executive functions. Our primary responsibility is to create a sense of mental and physical safety for those who depend on us, including our partners and children. When we are critical of our family members, no one feels secure. How do you feel when you are criticized? How do you think your family feels when you are angry?

Chronic mental and physical illnesses are rampant among teenagers. A 2013 paper published out of Indiana University School of Medicine surveyed forty-three pediatric hospitals across the United States.[13] The sample size was 3,752 patients, with a mean age of 13.5 years. From 2004 to 2010, admissions for chronic pain increased by 831 percent. What is stunning was that there was an average of ten diagnoses per patient. Doctors could not find a specific cause of the symptoms in most patients.

I gave a talk at a high school a few years ago and was told that over 350 of the 1,500 students had a chronic medical problem that had to be monitored. Eating disorders are increasing, even among males. Teen suicide is a serious problem. We have more resources and opportunities at our disposal than at any point in human history. Yet much of the population is miserable. We keep wringing our hands about the problem but are not coming up with actual solutions.

Much of our guidance stems from well-meaning parents who often criticize perceived flaws that might hinder our success. In other words, we are told what to do and what not to do from a young age. One classic example is sharing. At two years old, a child has no understanding of the word or the concept. We inform them that sharing is good and being selfish is bad. The child does not grasp what the parent is trying to convey, yet is repeatedly reprimanded, and everyone eventually becomes exhausted. A more straightforward and effective approach would be to consistently model generosity and politeness and avoid making the child feel guilty for their curiosity or desire to keep things for themselves. This is their natural inclination and drive. When punishment is involved, the child might feel like a bad person. Imposing adult values on a young child with an evolving brain is futile and leads to further issues.

If you are lucky and have the resources, you might be encouraged to live life to the fullest and succeed—to start organized sports early, travel the world, and be creative. There is no limit to what is possible. But that is also the problem. You can achieve many things, but you cannot outrun your mind. And when you accomplish what you think should bring peace of mind and you still feel unhappy, where do you go next? Then you feel trapped.

Most of us were raised with some level of criticism, but what if your parents were only supportive while also holding you to high standards across the board? Good grades, athleticism, attractiveness, a winning personality, an acceptable weight . . . How is this going to work? Not well. Inadvertently, standards—spoken or unspoken—create judgment. The higher the bar, the more self-criticism ensues when it isn't met. Then you have expectations from teachers, marketing, society, social media, and peers—all of which continually raise the ante. The result is rampant FOMO. The visual sensory input alone is perceived as a threat, not to mention the pressures to perform. The stage is set for threat physiology at a young age, and the effects are severe.

A 2022 study out of Spain examined obsessional intrusive thoughts (OITs) in forty-nine children ages eight to ten years, representing the first research of its kind in young children.[14] Results showed that 71 percent of the study's participants experienced OITs, with 29 percent reporting frequent, recent occurrences. Unlike adults, children primarily experienced thoughts as images rather than words, focusing on harm and doubt rather than contamination. Children with frequent OITs exhibited higher anxiety and OCD symptoms. Their coping strategies included negative self-appraisals, and they employed various control strategies, including thought suppression and seeking parental reassurance. Note that these approaches addressed the cognitive aspects of OIT, and the self-regulation of threat physiology wasn't mentioned.

A critical oversight in pediatric OCD research is physiological self-regulation strategies. While most of these children were found to be using thought suppression—a technique known to backfire—no body-based interventions, such as breathing exercises or mindfulness, were assessed. Safety-related thoughts dominated, with 46 percent of OITs involving harm, particularly fears about parents' safety, which suggests deep attachment concerns. Children rated their control strategies as only moderately successful (with an average rating of 43.84/100), highlighting the ineffectiveness of cognitive-only approaches. This research underscores the urgent need for developmentally appropriate interventions that incorporate somatic regulation techniques and address the mind-body connection in childhood anxiety and intrusive thoughts.

Instead of teaching our children to "be all that you can be," why not "just be"?

Your Programming Choice

Humans have a significant advantage over AI. We can self-program. We can choose what data to load into our nervous system—if the brain is online. Your programming is happening right now, whether you're aware of it or not. You have a significant choice to make right this second and every second going forward. Are you going to continue battling with the past, or are you going to choose how to program your nervous system? The only truly constructive question to ask yourself is, "How do I conduct myself today?" When you're not *reacting*, you can choose your programming inputs. RUTs overwhelm and disguise who you aspire to be, and also take your neocortex offline. Learn to recognize when you're reacting versus choosing what you do next. You can start proactively programming yourself right now.

Remember, your brain is constantly assessing your surroundings and adjusting to them. It changes structure, through neuroplasticity, according to its immediate needs. This is an automatic process, and to take charge of your ongoing brain construction, you must follow this basic sequence: awareness → separation → reprogramming. RUTs are a result of your lifetime of programming, and healing happens with reprogramming.

Awareness

Without awareness of where you already are, you cannot consciously evolve in a more positive direction. Whenever you're anxious or frustrated, these are signs that you're still stuck in the past, and your thinking brain is losing connectivity. You are reacting, which you are supposed to do in the face of physical threats. However, most mental threats are not immediately dangerous; the reactions are unnecessary and consume a lot of energy.

Awareness is at the center of healing and is what allows you to disconnect from your automatic survival reactions. The first step, though, is to recognize your survival reactions and become aware of your responses. The practical tools of thought separation, beginning with expressive writing, will be the topic of chapter 7.

Reprogramming

You didn't choose your initial programming, but you can now decide what happens next. (The exception to this is if you are in a situation of physical or emotional abuse, which might require outside intervention to restore you to a safe environment.) Your brain will evolve wherever you place your attention. There are countless ways to reprogram your brain, including various forms of play, pursuing your passions at work or at home, engaging in spiritual practices, helping someone in need or giving back to your community, practicing gratitude and compassion, or simply listening to a friend without judgment. The reprogramming possibilities are endless.

Another core strategy is committing to not discussing your pain—mental or physical—with anyone other than your health care providers. This is *especially* important when it comes to close family and friends. Your home and community are your best opportunities to feel safe. Make a point of nurturing them. Can you train yourself to walk in your front door with a smile, regardless of how you feel? If you are in a particularly bad mood, consider delaying going home until you can calm and recenter yourself.

When you complain, you are loading data into your brain that fires up the pain circuits, and also into those around you, especially your family. So, there are no shortcuts to this step. Just stop. Start training yourself to stop complaining now. It could take weeks to tone down your compulsion to talk repeatedly about your pain and anger, but you can resolve to stop right now. No one benefits from ongoing complaints. You'll learn about the power of expressive writing in chapter 7, and that is where you can safely express your negativity.

We often don't realize that mental pain is a bigger problem than physical pain. So not sharing your pain means:

- no complaining, unless you do so directly to the person who can resolve the issue, such as the person who is unwittingly causing you pain, or possibly a mental health professional
- no giving unasked-for advice—especially to your partner or children
- no criticism
- no gossiping
- stop searching for a cure for your pain

These simple rules are not as straightforward as they seem. As you start to cut out complaining from your day-to-day routine, you will realize how much of your life energy is being consumed by negativity. For many people, complaining is such a deeply ingrained behavioral pattern that it is difficult to change. Initially, you will fail frequently. That's okay, just be persistent. Within a couple of weeks, as the complaints become fewer and less intense, you'll notice many changes in the quality of your relationships. You will have more interesting conversations and more energy for enjoyable activities. You will also be more able to provide practical support to friends and family. It is not uncommon for a friendship to fade when one party stops discussing their pain or complaining about their life. Sharing negative emotions can provide a strong bond—but is it worth pursuing a bond that perpetuates pain?

Understandably, you might want to discuss your misery with anyone who will listen. When pain has engulfed your life, venting provides temporary relief and can bond you with other people who are suffering. But when you are busy complaining, think of everything else you are missing. What is this behavior doing to your pain circuits?

Research shows that belonging to a pain support group lessens your chances of healing. In these groups, there is often a lot of mutual complaining about families not paying enough attention, poor medical care, the doctors not listening, and failed procedures. They might all be legitimate complaints, and it is entirely understandable that you would want to share your troubles and get support.[15] But from a neuroplasticity viewpoint, it is a disaster. For the same reason, keeping a pain diary has also been shown to portend a worse prognosis.[16]

Another way to reinforce your pain circuits is to endlessly search for a cure. Why wouldn't you continue to seek a remedy for the distress, anxiety, and discomfort you are feeling? It is important to undergo a thorough medical workup to rule out anything serious; however, if the results are negative, it is advisable to stop obsessively searching for a cure. Between discussing your pain and medical care, researching online, seeking care, complaining to friends and family and fellow complainers, and implementing treatments, you are allowing a significant percentage of your consciousness to be occupied by pain. Neuroplastic changes are dictated by where you place your attention, so chronic complaining reinforces your pain circuits and allows them to become monstrous.

Summary

We are fundamentally shaped by every moment of our existence, particularly by childhood experiences that create unconscious patterns that govern our adult responses. Adverse experiences embed neural circuits that automatically trigger anxiety, anger, and destructive thought patterns throughout life. Research shows our unconscious mind processes millions of bits of information per second while consciousness handles only ten to fifty bits, which explains why changing ingrained patterns feels so difficult.

However, neuroplasticity offers profound hope. The exact brain mechanism that created our current programming can entirely reshape it. The key lies not in fighting old patterns, which only strengthens them, but in deliberately creating new neural circuits through focused attention and repeated practice.

The transformation process follows three steps: (1) awareness of current programming, (2) separation from reactive patterns, (3) deliberate reprogramming through new experiences. Rather than endlessly analyzing the past, we must learn the new language of an enjoyable life. Just as we can't learn French by fighting English, we can't heal by battling pain or anxiety.

Success requires consistently directing attention toward safety-generating activities that train your nervous system to feel secure. When your body feels genuinely safe, its natural healing capacity activates. The goal isn't to eliminate self-critical voices, but to learn to acknowledge them for what they are while choosing different actions, literally rewiring your brain to support the life you envision.

The biggest issue we're facing in the realm of mental health right now is that we don't know how to help people feel safe enough to heal. Learning to feel secure in the presence of perceived danger is the key. Get your brain online and repeatedly make safe choices from a connected brain. Train your brain to feel safe in the presence of unpleasant, dark emotions. Realize that your RUTs are thoughts rising from emotions. There is no physical danger; you are safe.

By the way, my golf game never improved, but I made a significant breakthrough in learning to let go of the score and enjoy my time with friends. Letting go is also a learned skill that helps to pave the way for positive reprogramming. In the next chapter, we will delve into the opposite of letting go: the need to take control.

CHAPTER 5

The Illusion of Control

If people are good only because they fear punishment, and hope for reward, then we are a sorry lot indeed.

—Widely attributed to Albert Einstein

Our need to control others, as part of our evolutionary programming, served our ancestors well when facing physical threats. Humans survived and evolved by seeking safety and using any means available to achieve it. We also became successful as a species by learning to work together in groups. Individuals were rewarded with a sense of safety when they shared similar characteristics with other members of the group. Anyone who was different was perceived as a threat—and was therefore mistreated or eliminated.

However, modern life presents a critical mismatch. Our ancient control mechanisms are now triggered by thoughts and emotions rather than saber-toothed tigers. Meanwhile, intolerance of differences runs deep in our evolutionary wiring and manifests at all levels of society. The result is a vicious cycle where the strategies that once ensured survival now create the suffering we're trying to escape.

RUTs are at the root of the problem. Although we can control many variables to live a functional life, there are many, if not more, that we cannot control—especially our thoughts and emotions. When we fail to control our inner world, we turn to external means of control.[1] As this does little to calm us down, we continue to redouble our efforts. Many of these efforts to exert control are damaging to ourselves and to others. Most of what drives these efforts are RUTs—thoughts that arise from perceived threats rather than actual ones.

Control feels like a solution because it provides temporary relief. And what viable alternative is there, when our physiology is wildly ringing the alarm? With an immediate threat, like fighting off an assault, taking immediate control is the solution. But what about disciplining a disruptive child? Or restricting one's diet to the point of anorexia?

Laboratory studies have shown that a sense of control lowers inflammatory markers.[2] Since it provides some relief, it reinforces the concept that control is effective, which keeps driving maladaptive control behaviors. Some of the most alarming consequences arise from trying to control basic human needs. We would never deny ourselves air, water, and the need to evacuate the bowel and bladder. Yet we often attempt to control sexuality and food intake. Someone with anorexia might experience an excellent mood while restricting their diet. Then, when they "fail," their mood will swing dramatically in the opposite direction. This creates an endless cycle of controlling behavior and threat physiology that is difficult to break.

Cutting is a method that some individuals use to inflict pain on themselves. By externalizing their mental pain, they create an illusion of control that provides a sense of comfort. Engaging in "active schadenfreude" or bullying activates the brain's pleasure circuits, allowing the bully to experience less pain temporarily, until they need their next fix.

As mentioned in chapter 3, the self-critical voice emanates from a dysregulated, hyperactivated sapiocortex, and self-inflicted schadenfreude occurs when the voice is validated. It never stops, and we engage in countless behaviors to silence it. We repeatedly attempt self-control and become determined to make a change. Or we set a high perfectionistic standard for ourselves and mentally berate ourselves if we don't meet it. Religions and belief systems of any kind are often frameworks that set these standards. Consequently, we might be overly strict with our children or spouse as we project our ideals onto them. When individual control strategies cannot provide lasting relief, we often project these same controlling impulses onto our relationships with others. Then no one feels safe.

This emphasis on external control is also culturally reinforced because every major institution is built around it, with hierarchical power structures rather than a system of self-regulation. Rigid standards are imposed in all organized religions. In authoritarian societies, entire groups of people are persecuted for their beliefs. Harsh disciplinary measures are common in school systems. The illusion of control as the solution to our problems is responsible for much human suffering, as we will explore further in this chapter.

If we were to create a culture of safety rather than of fear-based control, we could lower reactivity, allow productive conversations, encourage listening, and make problems more solvable. Collaboration versus competition would flip the paradigm of productivity. A foundational research paper titled "Self-Determination Theory and the Facilitation of Intrinsic Motivation, Social Development, and Well-Being" published in 2000 by Richard Ryan and Edward Deci presented three basic human needs: competence, autonomy, and relatedness.[3] When people act from their internal sense of values, they have more motivation, excitement, persistence, and enhanced performance. Note that money, often used as a form of control, is not the main driver. After a certain threshold of fair compensation, more money makes little difference to well-being.

Adaptive vs. Maladaptive Control

Let's define *control*. According to Merriam-Webster, it means "to exercise restraining or directing influence over" something. Anxiety is a danger signal that triggers our control mechanisms, which are part of our survival tool kit. It compels us to take protective action to remain safe. Each of us has a unique set of skills and resources to physically protect ourselves. Meanwhile, RUTs pose no immediate danger. These thoughts cannot physically hurt you. There is *nothing* there except your attachment to your thoughts. When you fight RUTs, you are swinging at thin air. When there is no physical threat, the solution to anxiety is to give up the need for control.

Repeated attempts to control the uncontrollable create a vicious cycle. Threat physiology (anxiety) triggers RUTs, which activate more threat physiology. As the balanced dance between the sympathetic and parasympathetic nervous systems fails, increased threat physiology—including the release of noradrenaline and dopamine—shuts down the PFC, which normally dampens threat responses. As this internal threat regulation system shuts down, we turn to external controls, which are ineffective, unsustainable, and trigger more RUTs and threat-related physiological responses. Sustained stress also compromises mitochondrial function, resulting in lower energy production.[4] With the energy for cognitive control depleted, we further rely on external controls.

There are two types of control: adaptive and maladaptive. Adaptive control is exerting a realistic influence on what is genuinely controllable;

regulating one's actions, choices, and responses to situations; and choosing wise actions while understanding what is not changeable.[5] Maladaptive control is a trap that results from attempting to control unwanted thoughts and emotions, often via misplaced attempts to control other people and external events. With this type of control, we are fighting internal experiences and constructs rather than understanding their true meaning and mechanisms. We are demanding certainty in inherently uncertain situations. Meanwhile, our altered thinking is blocking awareness of what we can and can't control.

We All Have Control Issues

How well do you like being told what to do, especially if it conflicts with your internal values? What about your children—how do you think they feel? Yet, parents, teachers, cultural codes, and societal norms raised most of us with rules of behavior. Many of these rules are arbitrary. For example, in the conservative boarding school I attended, we could not wear jeans, drink caffeinated beverages, listen to rock music, own a radio—the list goes on. At my medical school, a physician almost lost his job because he brought a coffee machine to work. If we step outside of norms, we are punished. If we stay within the prescribed lines, we are rewarded. Many of us are also held to high standards. Anything short of meeting these expectations is considered a failure. By the time we are adults, we have internalized these rules, standards, and expectations.

No one feels safe when being criticized, controlled, or treated with anger—whether it's coming from others or ourselves. Our nervous systems receive these negative inputs as threats, which in turn trigger our own controlling behaviors. It's a vicious loop. "She has control issues," you might gossip about someone. Guess what? Everyone has control issues to some degree. We were raised this way, held to rules and standards that often did more harm than good, and almost all of us continue to live under this over-controlling influence. Few of us know alternatives. Understanding why exerting control feels necessary (it's a survival sensation) helps explain why we persist with approaches that consistently fail. But perhaps the most damaging application of control occurs when we try to manage behavior through punishment—a strategy that not only fails to deter unwanted behavior but actively creates more of the problems it aims to solve.[6]

Why Punishment Backfires

When a child is upset and dysregulated, and therefore acting out, we must first ensure that they are safe. The best approach is to help them calm down by teaching and modeling self-calming skills to help regulate emotions. But what usually happens? We focus on behavior: "Stop that right now"; "You will be grounded for a week if you don't do as I say!" We employ many forms of control and discipline to stop unwanted behaviors. Our common approach to parenting, shaped by our own childhood experiences, emphasizes discipline and control while consistently focusing on outward behavior.

Expert hostage negotiators understand that this approach is ineffective. Instead, they consistently prioritize de-escalating the situation before attempting to resolve the issue. When was the last time you successfully solved anything with control during a heated argument? The person with more power might "win," but the relationship inevitably suffers.

This controlling mindset permeates our society, where harsh penalties such as lengthy prison sentences and the death penalty are prevalent. However, these extreme measures fail to deter negative behaviors effectively. Why? Because threat physiology is potent and behavioral interventions only create more threat, exacerbating the situation. For a while, a person might suppress their behavior out of fear, but fear raises their baseline threat level. How can this be sustainable over time?

The disturbing irony of attempting to suppress threat physiology through punishment is that many of the enforced standards of behavior are entirely arbitrary. They are based on one individual's, or group's, perception of reality. If someone violates or doesn't meet those rules, the rule setter criticizes or disciplines them. Control depends on a power balance. The more dependent a person is on another for basic needs, the greater the potential for abuse, which is a dynamic we'll revisit later in this chapter.

Let's take a look at how other common control strategies are failing us.

Three Types of External Control Strategies

When we are driven by anxiety and RUTs, there are endless ways we attempt to control and manipulate our environment to feel safe. The most common approaches fall within three basic strategies: escape, fix, and control. To some degree, and often unconsciously, most people resort to a combination of all three. Take a closer look and you'll quickly recognize that external controls cannot counteract internally generated pain.

Escape Strategies: Masking

Escape strategies include addictive behaviors that temporarily ease our mental pain while we are engaging in them. Although they provide short-term relief, these strategies are harmful across various areas of life. The examples are endless, including substance abuse of drugs and alcohol, gambling, overeating, overworking, and the excessive pursuit of sports or art at the expense of relationships and self-care. Engaging in these behaviors provides a brief escape from mental torment, but it's akin to taking a painkiller for a broken bone without setting it; the temporary relief masks the worsening underlying issue.

Extreme risk-taking sports embody another captivating form of masking behavior. While the admiring public witnesses extraordinary feats of human achievement, medical professionals confront the resulting consequences of head trauma, paralysis, long-term disability, and death. I have personal experience with this through my son, a national-level mogul and extreme skier. Over the years, he has witnessed the deaths of three fellow skiers and a coach who developed paraplegia. While the public celebrates these "adrenaline junkies," what we are truly witnessing is often a sophisticated form of self-medication. The rush of extreme danger temporarily drowns out the mental noise, but at what cost? This temporary relief comes with a genuine possibility of permanent consequences.

Other behaviors that people use to regulate RUTs and manage sensory input include compulsive habits. They provide soothing effects but might eventually become problematic. They often start innocently enough: nail-biting, skin-picking, hair-pulling, knuckle- and neck-cracking, and other repetitive actions. While these behaviors might begin as minor coping mechanisms that cause little disruption to your quality of life, they can reach a dangerous tipping point. For example, hair-pulling can lead to noticeable bald spots, and nail-biting could permanently damage the nail bed.

Let me share a story about a friend of mine, a retired physician. His experience illustrates how a seemingly harmless behavior can spiral completely out of control. He began picking at his skin after gardening one day. He had trimmed juniper bushes, which irritated his skin. Convinced he had multiple splinters embedded in his skin, he dismissed all rational explanations, including my argument that even if they were present, foreign objects work their way out within a few weeks. The picking persisted for over five years, and his perception escalated to where he believed he had shiny pink crystals under his skin.

Any suggestion from anyone that they weren't there would send this usually gentle person into a rage. It's important to understand that reasoning never works with these spinning thought patterns. While his behavior was driven by a deep-seated threat response, it manifested as a complex condition that likely involved other neurological factors.

As these self-soothing behaviors advance, they might become increasingly detached from reality—resulting, for example, in severe hoarding, repetitive stair walking, counting items, repeating phrases, embracing extreme religious views or other belief systems, arranging objects in specific patterns, and engaging in elaborate rituals. For some individuals, these behaviors are so subtle that they go unnoticed, while others might exhibit prominent and unusual behaviors that significantly disrupt their lives. Habits such as hair-pulling and nail-biting appear to be harmless, and indeed they might be. Or they can become intense attempts to mask and escape from RUTs.

Fix Strategies: Reassurance

Since RUTs often make us feel worthless and inferior, we try to combat them by "fixing" the perceived issue driving them. These efforts aim to refute negative thoughts by providing evidence to disprove them. We seek both validation and reassurance. This approach fails spectacularly because RUTs operate independently of evidence. Attempts at reassurance can inadvertently draw attention to these circuits and reinforce them.

The pursuit of reassurance takes many forms, such as accumulating more possessions, endlessly seeking medical cures despite extensive testing, obsessing over appearance, undergoing repeated cosmetic surgery, and chasing money, power, prestige, and accomplishments. There's over-exercising and hyper-focused bodybuilding, including the use of performance-enhancing drugs. The relentless pursuit of success can be driven by imposter syndrome and the constant need for reassurance to boost one's ego. None of these endeavors has a defined end point or limits on how long and how intensively they can be pursued. Let me share some stories that illustrate this endless need for reassurance.

A recent study of orthopedic surgery residents found that 73 percent experienced significant or intense impostor syndrome.[7] This is a psychological phenomenon in which individuals doubt their accomplishments and consistently fear being exposed as frauds. Although these surgery residents are among the highest achievers in medicine, they often feel that they are not worthy of their positions. One resident, despite scoring in the top quartile on all medical exams, constantly worried that she would be exposed as incompetent. Another, who had received awards for his surgical skills, spent hours each night reviewing basic procedures because he was convinced he was missing something fundamental that all the other residents understood. The study found that female residents were more than five times as likely to experience intense impostor syndrome as their male colleagues. It didn't matter how many surgeries they successfully performed or how many tests they passed—the feeling of inadequacy persisted.

Recently, I met with a friend's son, a competitive bodybuilder who had been banned for taking performance-enhancing substances. He felt devastated, as if his whole life had been taken away. He had reached out for some advice on how to handle his current legal situation. I was sitting across from him in a booth. His elbows were propped on the table—biceps so massive they sagged sideways, almost parallel with the surface. I had to make a concerted effort not to stare. Suddenly, he told me how small his arms felt and spent five minutes explaining how badly this made him feel. I couldn't believe it! Here was someone with biceps that dwarfed mine, yet in his mind, they weren't big enough. That's when I realized how serious body-image issues could be. No matter how much he tried to reassure himself through more training, his mind would never allow him to see reality.

I had a friend in her twenties with severe anorexia. Although she was conventionally attractive, she truly thought she was fat and extremely ugly. She couldn't find words to express her disgust. I asked her, "If one million people signed a statement of how attractive and fit you are, how would that work?" Her reply was, "They wouldn't really know who I am."

Over my thirty-two-year career as a spine surgeon, almost every patient I saw with ill-defined pain and anxiety believed that the prior clinicians had missed something. I would initially conduct any additional testing I thought necessary and then reassure them that everything was okay. But nothing I said would assuage their concerns. They would often seek additional medical testing, and the cycle would continue. The longer and more assertively I spoke to them, the more agitated they became.

The thought "My doctor is missing something because I'm in pain" becomes a repeatable neurological circuit that is no longer under cognitive control and won't shut down. Logic alone can't break it apart. The more you focus on these circuits, the stronger they become. I liken them to "dust devils" on the Midwest plains. These small but powerful mini tornadoes are unstoppable. The medical term for this phenomenon among patients is *injury conviction*.[8] I had first heard about injury conviction in medical school, but I did not understand its power and significance until I had patients of my own. Eventually, I understood that a patient's attachment to a diagnosis that wasn't there limited what I could do. I learned to let go of these patients, but I always felt a sense of sadness that I could not help them out of their predicament. (Chapter 7 will present the concept of cognitive fusion, which happens when your thoughts and self-concepts become so entangled that they become your identity. Any challenge to them feels like a personal assault.)

This problem has societal implications. The endless quest for answers is expensive. In the United States, 5 percent of patients consume 55 percent of health care dollars.[9] In the Washington Workers' Compensation system, 5 percent of patients consume 84 percent of resources.[10]

All of these individuals—the brilliant surgical residents with impostor syndrome, the massive bodybuilder who feels small, the person with an eating disorder who feels fat and ugly, and the patient with back pain seeking an elusive diagnosis—attempted to fix their anxiety and RUTs with external control strategies. It took me years to realize that the more I tried to reassure patients nothing was physically wrong with them, the more complicated our conversations became. I recognized that pushing back against their perception of reality was contributing to the problem. I also wanted to keep helping them, and it wasn't easy to let go.

Larger muscles, the bodybuilder believed, would silence his doubts. One more test would reveal the "real cause" of her pain, the patient insisted. The residents felt that additional studying and practice would finally make them feel like they belonged. The young woman with anorexia constantly strove for a better body. However, repetitive unwanted thoughts like these operate independently of evidence. They continue to spiral out of control, and efforts to refute them by proving them wrong are ineffective. As your threat physiology continues to spiral, there is an increasing possibility of self-destructing.

When even reassurance and external validation cannot quiet the internal storm, we reach for the most intensive strategy, which is direct control over ourselves, others, and our environment.

Direct Control Strategies

Direct attempts at control represent perhaps the most pervasive category of RUT-driven behaviors. The need for mental control serves as a primary driver of RUTs. When that strategy fails—as it so often does—we frequently resort to controlling our environment or behaviors. The need for mental control is impossible to satisfy, yet we keep trying.

Rigidity

Suppressing basic survival impulses creates havoc and often gets codified into rigid belief systems that demand impossible standards. Regardless of what you believe to be your truth, it is a function of your upbringing, culture, societal norms, and time period. What is true for you is not true for others. You have a right to live according to your own moral code, but you have no right to decide what is right for others. If your views become rigid, research suggests that you might not even be able to experience normal emotions, let alone recognize the needs of others.[11]

Of course, social mores allow us to coexist. Ancient codes of conduct such as the Ten Commandments have long served religious societies. The Babylonians introduced laws that regulated behavior with clearly defined penalties, compiled in Hammurabi's Code.[12] Most of these rules established reasonable boundaries that enabled people to integrate their lives, cooperate, defend themselves, and thrive.

But what happens when rules and laws reflect a dogmatic and punitive belief system, as is often seen in organized religion? I humbly acknowledge that a shared belief in a higher power can serve a greater good, and that a spiritual perspective can provide a solution for pain. However, the repetition of dogma leads people to confuse beliefs with facts that they insist others should live by as well. Instead of promoting acceptance and love, rigid belief systems take over. The focus shifts from fostering a haven of safety and peace to enforcing rules. This can happen in families, organizations, and entire societies. Even the feeling of anxiety, which is fundamental to our evolutionary wiring, can be labeled as wrong.

I met Kari in 2018 when she asked me to speak at her company's annual disability conference. I gave a presentation on the nature of chronic pain and the Dynamic Healing approaches to solving it. She contacted me about a year later and shared how excited she was: Having learned and applied the healing concepts I presented at the conference, she was experiencing significant improvements with her pain and repetitive thoughts. We have remained in close touch, and here is one of her emails after I had told her about the remarkable turnaround of a twenty-four-year-old gentleman who had broken out of his bipolar disorder, anxiety, major depression, and migratory pain:

> *Hi David, is this the young man with bipolar you mentioned during our call? What an incredible transformation! Because few children are taught how to process anxiety, they do the best they can on their own, often creating inaccurate perceptions of themselves and learning ineffective, often damaging behaviors to deal with it (the seven-year-old creates the fifty-year-old). Many parents haven't learned these [healing] skills and are trapped in their own heads with repetitive negative thoughts; therefore, they don't know how to teach their children. And the cycle of dysfunction continues . . .*
>
> *A little personal story here . . . My aunt gave me my grandmother's book of prayers. My grandma was an extremely anxious woman and pretty OCD. I was thumbing through her book and noticed that my grandma had written in the margins, underlined specific passages, and so on. In the section on anxiety, she had underlined several times that "anxiety is a sin." My poor grandmother thought she was a sinner her entire life because she was anxious! How awful!*

I am not suggesting that we should act on every basic impulse and permit children to act exactly as they please. The goal is to recognize these impulses for what they are, to separate our identity from these sensations, and to act in a way that best meets the needs of ourselves and those around us. It is the severe repression of the need to feel safe that leads to many bizarre behaviors. Perhaps nowhere is the futility of control more evident than when we attempt to suppress basic survival impulses. Consider sexuality—a drive so fundamental that attempting to control it often creates the very behaviors that religions and cultures are trying to prevent.

Suppressing Sexuality

When lifespans were much shorter there was no reason to delay childbearing, so early humans reproduced at much earlier ages than today. A strong sexual drive was (and still is) a sign of health. Men dominated the social hierarchy, while women were paired off based on position, power, and money. Basically, they were enslaved and could only hope for the kindness of their husbands. (It wasn't until the thirteenth century that the concept of chivalry and romance came into play.) Women had to start having babies at ages twelve to thirteen, and a lot of them. Infant mortality was high, and larger families had a higher chance of survival.

Compare that with the superimposed standard of one monogamous marriage for life, and anything else regarded as a sin. Consider also that, in our modern society, the onset of puberty and sexual activity typically begins several years before the legal age of consent. I am not advocating to change this social norm, which aims to protect young people who are not yet fully aware of the implications of sexual activity. I make this observation to show how the mismatch between our evolutionary wiring and modern social mores create a hotbed for RUTs. Consider the following story.

I spoke with a young man in his mid-twenties who has faced severe intrusive thoughts for many years. His father contacted me to see if I could help, after his son had undergone many unsuccessful and varying treatments. Initially, he wasn't open to my insights, as it has been his father's idea to start the conversation. I wasn't optimistic, but I have learned that patience and persistence are key. You cannot change a lifetime of programming in a few weeks. I did not hear from him for a couple of months, and his father reached out again. I insisted that his son call me. Surprisingly, he did, and this time he was open enough to begin using some of the basic tools.

After three months, he felt a slight shift in mood, and he began to engage more deeply. He made significant progress as he learned calming techniques, practiced awareness, understood the irrational nature of his thoughts, and retrained his nervous system. During our conversation, important details emerged about his strict Protestant upbringing, including his early exposure to a biblical passage that gave him obsessive thoughts.

He was about thirteen years old when he first encountered this text, which he shared with me:

> *Matthew 5: 27–29. "You have heard that it was said, 'You shall not commit adultery.' But I tell you that anyone who looks at a woman lustfully has already committed adultery with her in his heart. If your right eye causes you to stumble, gouge it out and throw it away. It is better for you to lose one part of your body than for your whole body to be thrown into hell."*
>
> *The passages from the Bible discuss a mere thought as equal to sin. This idea led me to struggle with intrusive thoughts and the associated anxiety. Since I felt condemned for the simple fact that intrusive thoughts arose—something I was utterly powerless to control—this resulted in tremendous agony, fear, doubt, and negative self-worth, causing me to believe I was in the wrong.*

The passage blew me away. I had heard it hundreds of times during my own religious upbringing, along with many other arbitrary rules that were impossible to keep. Not allowing yourself to think a lustful thought when you are thirteen is not only incredibly difficult but downright impossible when your body's hormones are raging. Talk about a textbook way of igniting unwanted thoughts.

A classmate of mine realized he was gay while in college. Guilt and relentless self-criticism plagued him, as he was constantly reminded by the church of the seriousness of this sin. He did not feel comfortable sharing his situation with anyone. He also endured abuse at home. While many other factors influence the onset of schizophrenia, his deep guilt was problematic, and he suffered a psychotic break. This challenging period endured for nearly five years before he emerged from this dark phase.

Stories like these show how impossible standards around natural impulses create relentless, obsessive thoughts about the very things they're trying to prevent. Punitive, shaming methods of control are unsustainable and almost always backfire—especially when trying to control RUTs.

Relationship Control

Consider the power dynamics in various types of relationships. The starker the power imbalance, the higher the potential for abuse. Consider the following escalating sequence of scenarios between you and another person:

A random stranger passing you in the street: You might throw an insult or even act aggressive toward them. They can simply walk away.

A bank or grocery store clerk: You might talk to them rudely and demand better service. They have to remain calm and professional with you, or else risk losing their job.

An employee or subordinate: You might become tough, assertive, or even overtly angry with them. Since they cannot afford to lose their job, which would hurt their career prospects and make it impossible to pay the rent (or mortgage), they might be willing to take a fair amount of abuse before deciding to quit.

A spouse or partner: You are emotionally volatile with your partner, with whom you have strong and complex bonds. Leaving a relationship isn't easy, especially if there is nowhere to go, so your partner might feel trapped and sustain significant abuse.

A child: When you are angry or aggressive with your child, they have little to no awareness of any other reality and depend entirely on you for their physical and emotional safety. The largest power imbalance occurs between a child and their adult caregiver. The potential for abuse is very high.

This sequence of scenarios charts an increasing potential for feeling or being trapped. Generally speaking, the most potent triggers of threat physiology are our family members, and most of our reactions and controlling behaviors are irrational responses based on past interactions and traumas.

We often believe that our children should be raised in a specific way, and we consider it our duty to instill our values in them and shape their character. In this context, there is constant criticism and discipline. But no one feels safe when faced with criticism. When you reflect on your childhood, how secure did you feel? Was being criticized and disciplined the norm for you? Do you know what safety feels like?

Verbal abuse is rampant in many families, as it was in mine. In the book *Verbal Abuse: Survivors Speak Out* by Patricia Evans, the stories are incredibly sad and all too common.[13] In how many people's lives are such circumstances the norm? The book is powerful but be warned that the stories of abuse are intense. Most of them are about women in abusive relationships. If you do read it, be prepared to be upset. It might help you realize that you are not alone, and prompt you to consider what you have normalized in your own relationships.

The primary responsibility of parents and caregivers should be to help their children feel safe. Yet, too many children become targets of a powerfully dysregulated nervous system and become dysregulated themselves for life. It is disturbing that so many people end up this situation and I continue to feel perplexed and disturbed by this trend.

One issue is that families often spend long periods in close proximity, and parents carry reactive patterns from their family backgrounds. This is why a significant percentage of people who abuse others were themselves abused. The essence of abuse is a lack of awareness of others' needs. Anger blocks awareness. Thus, the abuser might not realize the impact they are having on those who depend on them for safety. Additionally, it is easier to become angry when under significant stress. In an abusive household, no one feels safe.

Another factor is that most workers in America either dislike or hate their jobs, which isn't a great way for people to spend the majority of their waking hours. When you return home, you might vent your frustrations to your family, making them feeling unsafe. Between work and family, over 50 percent of parents feel stressed and often blame their children.[14] Children cannot be less stressed than their parents, and the bidirectional triggers of threat physiology becomes toxic. Rather than using calming tools, parents often reach for punitive controls.

What do you want for your life? What do you want for your family, friends, and coworkers? You wish to feel safe and to create an environment where they, too, feel safe—both mentally and physically. For parents, providing a safe environment is fundamental to raising healthy children. Yet, how often is this our focus? Instead, how often do we focus on behavior, achievements, and outward appearances? How often do we use the critical voice? This is a surefire driver of threat physiology and RUTs.

When neither individual control nor relationship control behaviors can provide lasting relief, we reach the most desperate level: extreme control strategies, via self-destruction. This includes both self-sabotage (destroying what we've built) and suicide (ending the life that has trapped us in uncontrollable threat physiology).

Extreme Control: Self-Destruction

We have many ways of self-destructing. Self-sabotaging behaviors include procrastination, being late for critical appointments, knowingly taking on more than we are able to deliver, and engaging in irrational behavior—such as having affairs with subordinates, damaging long-term friendships with insults, and embezzling from your employer. When your brain is used to struggling amid chaos, it is familiar territory. Success feels unfamiliar and causes anxiety. Then the anxiety downregulates your thinking brain and better judgment. Paradoxically, self-sabotage can feel like control over an uncomfortable situation. Think of the times when anxiety has led you to engage in self-sabotaging behaviors. What set the stage for your anxiety, and what were the consequences of your actions?

Self-destruction might seem counterintuitive as a control strategy, but it follows the same logic as all control behaviors. When we can't control our internal experience, we'll take control in any way we can—even if it means destroying what we've built. Consider the number of high-profile people who have had an affair with a subordinate and ended up losing their careers; prominent religious leaders who have committed improprieties or abuse; superstar athletes, actors, and musicians who have self-destructed in various ways. All of these people have achieved far more than what most of us can hope for. Why blow up what they've worked so hard to achieve?

Each case is unique and multifaceted, but there is a common denominator: Success creates anxiety. The more successful you are—in terms of power, wealth, and status—the more there is to lose, and the more social pressure you feel to keep succeeding. At a certain point, an inflamed nervous system might unconsciously choose familiar chaos and self-destruction over continued achievement. Also, I have observed that many high-achieving people are driven by RUTs, and are constantly seeking validation and escape from the self-critical voice. But no one can outrun their mind.

Suicide represents the highest level of self-destruction—the most extreme manifestation of behavior driven by RUTs. It is the ultimate attempt at control. When an individual feels trapped with no conceivable escape, suicide appears as the only solution to silence unwanted thoughts.

You can feel trapped by mental pain from RUTs, physical pain, relationships, finances, or progressive illness. The situation worsens when you're not heard, dismissed by medical professionals, or unsure that the suffering will ever end. Scientific evidence shows a direct link between ruminating thoughts and suicide. These repetitive unwanted thoughts create a mental prison more confining than any physical barrier.[15] The prevalence of suicide among medical professionals is alarming. I've lost over twenty colleagues to suicide, including a good friend and spine surgeon who was assisting me on a complex spine operation. He said he had an appointment and had to leave. He shook my hand, walked out of the operating room, and took his life.

Counterintuitively, once a person has made a suicide plan, their mood often improves. This is similar to a person with anorexia whose extreme dietary restrictions make them feel better—more in control. Thus, a lift in mood can be a worrisome sign that someone is resorting to an extreme control measure that calls for intervention. People need to understand that suicide is a completely unnecessary way to escape the trap of RUTs. There are consistently effective paths to healing that can bring you back to a life of your choosing.

Given that control-based approaches to stopping negative behaviors so frequently backfire, what's the alternative? The answer can be found in understanding how our nervous system works. Instead of fighting our physiology, we can work with it through Dynamic Healing—a framework that addresses the root cause of our struggles rather than just managing symptoms. This approach recognizes three fundamental components that determine whether we feel safe or threatened.

Dynamic Healing: Safety Instead of Control

When stress-driven thoughts overwhelm you, the definitive solution is to restore your physiology to a state of safety. The Dynamic Healing framework evolved out of the informal scientific study group that began with a phone conversation with Dr. Stephen Porges. Building on a foundation of evolutionary biology, Stephen and his wife, Sue Carter, presented a basic principle: Living creatures continuously gather information, process it, and respond in ways that optimize survival. This happens through three interconnected systems that determine whether we feel safe or threatened:

Input represents everything flowing into your nervous system—stress from work, relationship conflicts, financial pressure, physical pain, even positive changes like promotions or new homes. Your body collects this sensory data like a sophisticated radar system, constantly scanning for potential threats.

Processing occurs in your nervous system, which analyzes this flood of information faster than any computer, asking one crucial question: "Am I safe or in danger?" This analysis happens below conscious awareness, but it determines everything about how you feel and function.

Output is your body's response—either shifting into safety mode where healing, creativity, and connection flourish, or threat mode where muscles tighten, thinking becomes cloudy, and chronic symptoms emerge.

Your physiological state depends entirely on the dynamic interaction between your life stresses and your coping resources, which constantly fluctuate between safety and threat. When stress exceeds your capacity to handle it, your nervous system tips into threat physiology—the root cause of most chronic illness, anxiety, and unwanted thoughts. Mainstream medicine focuses on suppressing symptoms, which is like trying to extinguish an oil well fire with water. The flames keep raging because the fuel source—threat physiology—remains untouched.

Root Causes of Chronic Illness

Doctors are largely dedicated to their patients and their well-being. However, the modern medical system often prevents doctors from having sufficient time to communicate effectively with their patients. How can we understand your living situation and the challenges you face? Often, people become ill in the backdrop of unusual stresses or significant life changes. Even positive ones—such as getting married, moving to a better job, having a child, or building a dream home—have a significant impact.

We don't have time to get to know you. What coping skills do you possess? Are we teaching you better ones? Do you feel supported by your medical team? Do you feel heard? Is your nervous system calm or hypersensitive? Are you sleeping? Do you exercise? What is your diet? Did you have a chaotic upbringing? What is your physiological state? What calming strategies do you use? Is your blood pressure elevated? Does your heart race? Do you experience palpitations at night when trying to fall asleep and relax? Are you engaging in addictive behaviors to calm down or mask symptoms? What control strategies are you using? All of these factors affect the state of your nervous system.

Symptoms are your body's way of alerting you that something is wrong. RUTs are symptoms that are also a source of threat. They are only resolved by addressing the root cause. Mainstream medicine's focus on isolated symptoms and interventions does not work. Chronic illness is a complex systems problem that affects your entire physiology. You must address all relevant variables to restore a state of safety.

Let's say you spot a wildfire and call 911. The first fire chief to arrive on the scene is the one in charge and sets up the base of operations. They must coordinate efforts. Extinguishing the blaze requires assessing the situation, containing it, and neutralizing or removing its fuel source. It requires multiple different strategies, depending on the height of the flames, local terrain, weather, and many other factors. For example, fire travels more quickly up a steep hillside, especially when it is dry and fanned by a strong wind. Compare that with a brush fire on flat land, without wind, and with moisture in the air.

Multiple interventions for containing and extinguishing the fire must be implemented simultaneously. Similarly, when you are in a state of inflammatory threat physiology, you must become the fire chief who takes charge of your care. Instead of deploying isolated controls that only temporarily mask the larger problem, you need to understand the bigger picture and make a coordinated plan.

Summary

Suppressing threat physiology—whether through mental control or behavioral interventions—perpetuates and exacerbates the problems it aims to resolve. When we can't manage our internal experience, we often attempt to control external factors and conditions, leading to destructive cycles that further trap us in a state of threat. A viable alternative is learning how to generate safety cues that interrupt and reverse this cycle, restoring us to a state of safety.

A common control strategy is to suppress outward behavior through criticism, discipline, and punishment. But these methods backfire spectacularly because they create more threat, not less—it's like throwing oil onto a fire. When we feel unsafe, our thinking brain shuts down, muscles tighten, and we literally cannot think clearly. The only way out is to de-escalate our threat physiology before attempting to solve the problem.

Control-based systems become increasingly harmful as power imbalances grow—from the random interaction of two strangers (minimal power differential) to a parent-child relationship (maximum power differential). Power imbalances and controlling mindsets permeate modern society: in families that prioritize model behavior and high performance over feelings of safety, in religious organizations that prioritize dogma and rules over spiritual connection, in schools that prioritize rankings over individual needs, in workplaces that motivate employees with fear and competition, in criminal justice systems that impose harsh penalties that don't deter crime—the list is endless.

Dynamic Healing offers a highly effective systematic alternative to control strategies, through three interconnected pillars: input, processing, and output. Our physiological state depends on the ongoing dynamic interaction between our stressors and coping resources. When stress exceeds capacity, our nervous system tips into threat physiology—the root cause of most chronic illness, anxiety, and unwanted thoughts. The solution isn't to exert more control but to create the conditions for safety. When we feel safe, our thinking brain functions optimally—we can listen, learn, connect, and solve problems creatively. True healing requires regulating the nervous system, restoring balance between the sympathetic and parasympathetic nervous systems, and cultivating safety physiology.

Dynamic Healing isn't just another healing tool but a conceptual model of care that represents a fundamental shift from fighting our physiology to working with it. Instead of asking, "How can I control this?" we ask, "How can I feel safe?" This simple reframing changes everything, because safety is the natural state where healing, creativity, and connection flourish.

In the next part of the book, I will lay out the process of healing that consists of four parts. You'll use all of them throughout your day.

Part Three

Your Healing Journey

CHAPTER 6

A Fourfold Path to Transcending RUTs

Are you more scared of failure, or not knowing how wildly successful your life could've been?

—Unknown

Imagine taking a much-anticipated camping trip to the mountains. The scenery is breathtaking. You hop onto a small fishing boat on a lake surrounded by high, rocky peaks, and the water is crystal clear. What a magnificent spot to relax and take it all in. You set out to enjoy the evening and watch the sunset. But there is a problem. Halfway across the lake, you notice a significant leak in the bottom of the boat, and you only have a small bucket to bail out the water. No matter how hard you bail, more water comes rushing in, and soon you can barely keep the boat afloat. You are so focused on the hole and trying to stay afloat that you have no capacity to enjoy the gorgeous surroundings. Your weekend getaway in the mountains has been ruined; you just want to get back to shore.

The boat is your defense (survival physiology) that keeps you afloat amid life's challenges. The hole is the connection of your conscious brain to your threat physiology and taking it personally. Your survival quartet of anxiety, envy, anger, and schadenfreude is the water pouring in. Counteracting it with your mind is futile, consumes all of your attention, and burns up a lot of energy. In this state of affairs, you can't possibly look up to appreciate the life you have, let alone envision the life you want. Instead of trying to bail out the water as fast as it's coming in, there are two things you can do: (1) plug the hole, and (2) enjoy the scenery. These are two parts of a linked skill set, and they are equally important.

We commonly engage in endless activities to lead fulfilling, happy lives, but instead of enjoying these activities, we often spend too much of our time trying to solve problems in ineffective ways. We feel stressed and think that fewer problems would make us happier. That might be partially true, but problems never stop arising. Life is full of challenges, both expected and unexpected. What about RUTs? They aren't going away either. But we can learn strategies for plugging the leak when it springs, so we can get back to more restorative and creative endeavors. Envision yourself sitting in the middle of the lake, bobbing peacefully in a boat that isn't leaking. Now you can sit back and replenish your energies for whatever lies ahead.

From early childhood, many of us are stuck in survival mode, and as life keeps coming at us, we endlessly try to keep our heads above the water. Where did the fun go? At what point in our lives were we taught the skills to calm and redirect our nervous systems? When were we taught to nurture joy? How long can we stay in survival mode before we buckle?

Daniel Coyle's *The Talent Code* has helped many of my patients to understand the neuroplastic aspects of healing. The same principles that apply to a specific type of talent apply to navigating life. The most influential people, Coyle notes, make their contributions before the age of forty-five. I found this curious. Why would people give up on their dreams at midlife? How do we get worn down so early? Why do so many of us end up spending our lives bailing water from a leaky vessel instead of patching up the hole and enjoying the journey? Because we have inadvertently become experts at suffering.

When I was young, I often heard my elders describe a friend or family member as having a nervous breakdown. It almost sounded like a rite of passage for adults in middle age. I did not grasp how serious it could be. Nervous breakdowns now appear to be more prevalent among younger people—those in their teens, twenties, and thirties.

What makes RUTs and the resultant anxiety more powerful is our ongoing resistance to them, which causes what Coyle calls deep learning. Interacting with new information in a complex way stimulates deep learning, which is the foundational step in creating genius. Correcting mistakes is a basic form of this process. However, it also strikes me that battling our thoughts achieves the same effect. Because we dislike them, we use energy trying to correct or suppress them. We become geniuses at feeling mental pain. People spend nowhere near as much energy embracing positive inputs.

Instead of noticing and interpreting our anxiety as an essential tool in our survival toolbox, we understandably do everything possible to escape or suppress it, and this is precisely what grants it power. Understanding how we became experts at suffering (and stopped pursuing our dreams) points us toward the solution.

The Fourfold Path: From Reactive to Creative

The paradigm shift is captured by a simple play on words: from *reactive* to *creative*. Take the *C* from the middle of *reactive* and place it first to get *creative*. This shift represents the journey from automatic survival responses to conscious, creative engagement with life.

When you're reactive, you're responding to something from the past, stuck in survival mode with your thinking brain offline and no actual choice available. When you're creative, you're present, aware, and able to direct your energy consciously toward what you want to create. To transition from reacting to creating, you need to learn skills to calm your body and reroute your nervous system. These skills can be grouped into four healing approaches, and each is as equally important as the other.

What follows is not a sequential program, but an integrated approach—four paths to healing that eventually merge into one continuous process. When you are learning to play an instrument or a sport, you must first learn the individual components and practice until you can flow them together naturally and intuitively. The same principle applies to the following four elements of healing:

- separating your identity from survival reactions by disengaging from your thoughts
- calming your physiology, including your nervous system, to create safety
- softening your concept of self, or ego
- redirecting attention toward creativity and the life you actually want

Separating yourself from your survival reactions is foundational to calming your body to heal your mind. Because your identity mainly consists of thoughts woven into concepts and stories that you believe about yourself, detaching from your thoughts is a crucial first step. It's nearly impossible to heal without engaging in some version of thought separation. The other three approaches are ways of creating safety. Let's briefly examine each of these four elements to understand how they work together to plug the leak and restore your capacity to enjoy the journey.

Separate from Your Thoughts

It is well documented that we cannot control our thoughts, and that we have no natural protection from unpleasant thoughts or emotional pain. As discussed in the last chapter, our need for mental control causes a great deal of havoc. The only alternative is to notice our thoughts and intentionally separate from them. Some techniques include:

Expressive writing: Recording your thoughts and then immediately destroying the paper helps you to separate those thoughts from yourself, visually and physically.

Active meditation and mindfulness exercises: Focusing on immediate physical sensations redirects your attention from RUTs. Instead of fighting your thoughts, you are switching sensory inputs.

Awareness: As you develop your ability to separate from your thoughts, you can nurture awareness of the links between your reactions and your thoughts. Awareness both breaks these links to the reactions that bind you to the past, and also connects you to creativity, which allows you to move forward. You cannot move forward without breaking free from the past.

We will explore these methods of thought separation in greater depth in the next chapter.

Calm Your Physiology ("Turn Down the Heat")

Healing occurs when you feel safe. In the wild, anger might help an animal defend itself when physically threatened, then quickly subside once a sense of safety is restored. Reactive anger in this context is limited to when it is necessary. However, RUTs are not physically threatening; they create an illusion of danger and are relentless. The anger reaction to RUTs will not make you or anyone around you feel safe.

Chapter 8 will cover methods for calming your stress physiology. In dealing with anxiety and anger, you must utilize strategies from all aspects of the Dynamic Healing framework—being mindful of the input, processing, and output elements of the nervous system. Again, you cannot eliminate or conquer a negative thought or emotion. Instead, you can learn to coexist with it, depersonalize it, cognitively separate from it, and even appreciate it as a survival tool. Calming your physiology—literally turning down the heat of inflammation throughout your body—is the tipping point for healing from any chronic illness.

Soften Your Ego

The third element of this process addresses one of the biggest obstacles to healing: the ego. You might be thinking, "What do you mean, 'soften my ego'? Everyone needs a strong ego." Really? Why? The ego is essentially a defense mechanism that's deployed to help you feel better about yourself and present yourself in a favorable light to others. Your ego relies on the judgments and opinions of others, leaving you at their mercy. It develops into self-judgment. Defending the ego is a core driver of RUTs, and it needlessly consumes a lot of precious energy.

The ego relies on cognitive distortions and labels. In other words, many elements of your sense of identity are cognitive distortions. When you are defending your ego, you are using distortions to reinforce distortions and create more distortions. As your efforts to strengthen your ego take you down a dark alley, you double down and develop mental rigidity. Then you are stuck, and breaking through this barrier of mental rigidity is the greatest obstacle to healing. As we will see in chapter 9, cultivating awareness and compassion can soften your ego and free you from its dark confines.

Connect to Creativity

The final and most significant component of healing is redirecting attention to more enjoyable, functional, and solution-focused neural circuits. This becomes increasingly possible as you create more space for new inputs and processing changes. Simply put, real healing occurs as you nurture and live the life you want. You can apply creativity to every aspect of your life, positive and negative. Life is full of challenges, and it always will be. Fully engaging in problem-solving with a creative approach is essential to restoring balance to your physiology and improving your quality of life. Often, we spend too much time feeling sorry for ourselves instead of redirecting our focus on solutions. The great news is that once you can consistently connect to creativity, your brain will continue to change in the direction of your choice through the power of neuroplasticity. Creative problem-solving builds newer, more functional circuits in your brain, but this can only happen when you feel safe.

Principles for Application of These Steps

Applying any one of these four healing approaches will not cause your RUTs and negative emotions to disappear into thin air forever. Your identity is intertwined with them because a lifetime of programming has permanently embedded them in your brain. Significant healing can only happen with increased mastery of these skills, to the point where you can integrate them all, simultaneously, into your daily life. They are all a part of the Dynamic Healing framework—a different way of navigating your life, rather than a linear roadmap to a final destination.

The goal is not to feel safe and content most or all of the time. This expectation is a trap. At any moment, a negative input might destabilize you and pull you out of a state of safety physiology; life is full of mishaps, obstacles, and adversity. If you are expecting to achieve a state of ongoing peace and harmony, you will be frustrated at the first setback. This will only further inflame your threat physiology. But when you view adversity as inevitable, you can use it to practice your skills. You learn more by "failing" and getting back on your feet than by trying to maintain constant peace.

Please don't rush through the practical applications of the fourfold path and treat them like it's work. *Working at healing* is an oxymoron. That would be like Sisyphus, the king in Greek mythology who was punished by the gods to push a large boulder up a hill. Each time he neared the top, it would roll back down. The gods condemned him to perform this task forever. Instead, focus on learning and mastering skills, not on the outcome. As you learn how to feel safe, your body will heal itself. You are learning how to engage fully in your own life. Engage with a sense of curiosity, gratitude, openness to new ideas, spirituality, and play. Play, as we will see in chapter

10, is the ultimate haven of safety. The more you can enter this mindset, the better.

More health care practitioners are incorporating many of the concepts outlined in this book into clinical care. It is important to find a program that you understand and enjoy. But, whichever one you choose, stick with one—jumping around is counterproductive. Spend only about ten to twenty minutes a day on a course, and maybe up to an hour total learning more about the healing process from any source that works within the principles of Dynamic Healing. Use the rest of the day to practice. The focus must be on learning skills, as opposed to monitoring your progress. There is rarely a direct cause and effect for an isolated treatment.

Over the course of fifteen years, in the midst of my busy clinical practice, I developed a set of resources and have made them available in my book *Back in Control* and on www.backincontrol.com. The latest rendition of my Direct Your Own Care (DOC) Journey course is available at www.thedoc-journey.com. I initially wrote *Back in Control* to explain the healing concepts in enough detail to make a clinical impact, but I quickly realized I needed to create an action plan, too. When patients implemented the concepts in an action plan, they began to heal consistently. Consistent engagement in the healing process predicted success, and many patients saw big improvements in their physical and mental health within six months. Since I stepped down from clinical practice, I no longer offer medical advice, but I currently coach twice a week in a group setting for an hour.

Figure out which methods of calming your body and healing your mind work best for you. The four parts of healing that I've outlined in the next four chapters are foundational to—not a substitute for—your mental health care.

Summary

Most of us spend our lives in an exhausting battle, attempting to use our conscious minds to tame our unconscious survival reactions. We suppress anxiety, wrestle with anger, and try to intellectually solve our way out of suffering. We are too busy trying to bail ourselves out of a sinking boat to pause and see that there's a solution: plug the leak, catch our breath, and enjoy the view.

Paradoxically, the way to solve the unsolvable is to stop trying to solve it. Humans face a unique evolutionary predicament—while animals can escape physical threats in the wild, we cannot escape our thoughts in social captivity. We've weaponized survival mechanisms against mental phenomena that exist only in our minds, creating chronic threat physiology that fuels most illness and suffering. We are fighting the invisible enemy of our thoughts, and we are the ones who gave power to them.

The solution emerges through the Dynamic Healing framework, which recognizes that all living creatures continuously gather information (input), process it through their nervous systems (processing), and respond by shifting into either safety or threat mode (output). Your physiological state depends entirely on this dynamic interaction between your life stresses and your coping resources.

The fourfold path works within this framework: separating identity from survival reactions, calming the nervous system to create safety, softening ego defenses, and reconnecting to creativity to rebuild the brain. These elements eventually merge into one fluid process centered on awareness—the tool that transforms us from reactive to creative. Soon, with the leak plugged and your boat intact, you'll finally be free to sit back and enjoy the magnificent view that was always there.

CHAPTER 7

Separate from Your Thoughts

Between stimulus and response, there is a space. In that space lies our freedom and our power to choose our response. In our response lies our growth and our happiness.

—VIKTOR E. FRANKL

"You are not your thoughts." This phrase, commonly attributed to Viktor Frankl, rings hollow because it feels like we *are* our thoughts. There is a physiological reason for this feeling: cognitive fusion. *Cognitive fusion* refers to becoming so entangled in thoughts, beliefs, or judgments (in the absence of objectivity) that it leads to rigid identification with them.[1] We automatically identify with our mental content—taking our thoughts to represent us rather than recognizing them as temporary mental events. Identification occurs with essentially all our thoughts—both positive (I'm competent) and negative (I'm a loser). The process is that a thought arises → we take it personally → it becomes part of our identity → we defend it as "truth." The more embedded it becomes in our nervous system, the harder we defend it.

Identity and *ego* are closely related terms, and in this book I am using them interchangeably. I refer to them to describe the process of building and defending a sense of self against perceived threats. There are varying definitions of ego, but it is essentially a summation of our thoughts and self-concepts that fuse with our identity. Our ego defines our place in the world. We work hard to monitor and guide our thinking to create what we consider an acceptable image for the world and ourselves. The more fiercely we defend our ego, the less mental flexibility we have. Ego is cognitive fusion.

Arguably, the strongest source of RUTs is taking our survival sensations personally. A necessary step is understanding that our survival physiology is there to protect us, but it is not who we are. Breaking up cognitive fusion separates us from these unpleasant or threatening sensations. As we separate from our RUTs, we are creating space for new circuits to develop and flourish.

The Neurochemistry of Cognitive Fusion

The development of human language enabled the PFC to create abstract self-concepts—mental stories about who we are. When we are not focused on external stimuli, our brain's default mode automatically activates self-referential thinking, continuously reinforcing these identity narratives. This creates a neurological trap: When our fused identity feels threatened, the amygdala responds exactly as if it were in physical danger, triggering threat physiology. For example, our boss's criticism of our work becomes the neurological equivalent of a bear attack. Each time we react to a thought as definitively ours (e.g., "I am a failure at my job") rather than as a transient mental event, we strengthen the neural circuits connecting that thought to our identity.

The resulting cascade of stress hormones and reactions—cortisol, adrenaline, excitatory neurotransmitters, and inflammatory responses—damages both mental and physical health. This explains why identity-based conflicts feel so overwhelming and why cognitive approaches to appeasement often fail. We're not dealing with logical problems but with ancient survival circuitry that treats threats to our self-image as existential emergencies requiring immediate defensive action. Why did we need this extreme threat response? It provided humans an evolutionary advantage because quick categorization and identity formation aided survival in groups. But in the modern world, what once aided survival now creates suffering through rigid self-concepts.

Language is central to forming identity or ego. In cognitive fusion, we go from "I am running" (temporary action) to "I am a runner" (fixed identity). Language creates the capacity for abstract self-concepts. Research has shown that about 90 percent of our thoughts are factually wrong, and most worries don't materialize. Our unconscious brain is geared toward detecting threats as we seek safety. We have all heard the phrase, "It is better to be safe than sorry." Our survival instincts could not agree more, so we produce a barrage of defensive thoughts, whether expressed or suppressed, and they become embedded in our concept of self (ego).

In chapter 9, we will explore the parallel development of the ego and mental rigidity, and why softening the ego is essential for healing. There are effective ways to accomplish this once you understand the nature of the problem. The first step, however, is to separate your identity from your survival physiology—which, thanks to cognitive fusion, means you must separate your concept of self from your thoughts.

A Word of Caution

Ego and mental rigidity developed for a reason. In nature, wild animals are always in some state of alertness. When a physical threat arises, they typically face a specific foe or situation, using their defensive skills to escape or neutralize the threat. If they don't succeed, they are injured or killed. Whatever happens, they face a defined scenario and outcome. Since human physiology responds to unpleasant thoughts similarly to physical threats, humans face an endless number of perceived threats that often have no connection to physical reality. You can't fight this war against an invisible internal enemy with seemingly limitless ammunition. An important step is to learn to give up the fight.

What you are not giving up on is living your life on your own terms. Instead of having to face down your fears like a cornered animal, you can transcend them. You can recognize them for what they are and consciously move yourself out of their firing range and move forward with your life. But you must possess the skills to accomplish this. Each of us learns in our own way and at our own pace. The secret is an openness to learning, persistence, and a desire to live your life instead of fighting it.

Since your thoughts and identity are already tightly fused together, separation exercises are necessary, and healing cannot happen until you create space between them. In my surgical practice, the first steps I would recommend to my patients were to (1) read *Back in Control*, (2) begin expressive writing, (3) come back in two weeks to discuss the next steps. On the return visit, I could immediately tell if they had started the expressive writing. Some patients noticed an almost immediate decrease in pain and improvement in mood. If they did not initially feel better, they felt a shift that they couldn't describe. Some found the exercise to be a little overwhelming, so we would set aside expressive writing and work on relaxation tools for a while. A few patients experienced dramatic relief right from the start. Many patients felt enough of an improvement that they thought expressive writing was a solution. I reminded them that it was only the starting point, but a necessary one.

If you experience some initial worsening of anxiety and RUTs as you start expressive writing, it is generally not a problem; it is actually an indicator that change is taking place. However, if this exercise starts to feel overwhelming, stop. Jump ahead to the next chapter (chapter 8) and use those calming strategies to lower your threat physiology. At any point on this healing journey, if your anxiety becomes overwhelming, stop and regroup with calming exercises before moving on. There is no hurry, and it is important to feel safe at every point along the way.

The strategies for thought separation presented below have a 5 to 15 percent chance of causing you to initially experience more anxiety.[2] After observing this a few times, I switched to recommending writing in stream of consciousness (writing out all thoughts—good, bad, and neutral) instead of writing out negative thoughts specifically. I have seen essentially no problems with this approach. It is also effective. Feeling emotionally unstable doesn't mean you should not pursue the expressive writing process, but to proceed with caution. If you have a major mental health diagnosis—such as OCD, major depression, severe anxiety, bipolar disorder, schizophrenia, suicidal thoughts, or another significant diagnosis—please check in with your mental health professional. If you currently work with a therapist or trusted mental health support, let them know you are pursuing this path. These concepts and tools are intended to add depth to your usual care, not to serve as a substitute.

If you feel stable enough after using the calming tools in the first part of chapter 8, you can try expressive writing again, but proceed slowly. Moving through the learning process too quickly can be overwhelming and counterproductive. The more you can bring a sense of curiosity and playfulness to the process, the better. This should not feel like work or a big project. After you understand the basic concepts outlined in this book, you only need to spend about ten to twenty minutes a day learning tools and strategies to lower stress physiology and nurture safety. Thought separation exercises should be done daily for just a few minutes, although you might decide to write for a long time when challenges seem insurmountable. As you incorporate these healing strategies into your daily routine, you'll be able to use these them for the rest of your life—whenever you need to calm and recenter yourself, reconnect to curiosity and creativity, and regain perspective.

Why Thought Suppression Backfires

Remember the ironic effect and Daniel Wegner's polar bear experiment in chapter 1? The harder you try not to think about something, the more it dominates your mind. This isn't a character flaw but simply how the brain works, as revealed by decades of research. When you suppress a thought, your brain engages two competing systems: The "operating process" works overtime to push away unwanted thoughts, while the "monitoring process" continuously scans to check whether the forbidden thought has returned—keeping the unwanted content at the forefront of consciousness. When stress depletes mental resources, the operating process fails while monitoring continues. Result? Unwanted thoughts become more prominent than before suppression began.

Brain imaging confirms this paradox. Even when people report successfully avoiding thoughts, research shows increased unconscious activation of that exact content. Suppressed thoughts become increasingly primed and accessible, ready to burst into consciousness. This internal battle consumes energy. Functional MRI studies show thought suppression simultaneously activates cognitive control regions while increasing amygdala activity—your brain's threat center.[3] As Dr. James Pennebaker observed, keeping parts of ourselves hidden requires "significant metabolic and cognitive energy." This constant suppression depletes working memory, impairs problem-solving, and creates the mental equivalent of holding a beach ball underwater. Inevitably you'll fatigue.[4]

The Physical Toll

The consequences of suppression and rumination extend beyond mental fatigue. Research has established clear links between thought suppression and measurable physical damage. Studies of nearly 300 healthy adults found that negative, repetitive thoughts directly predicted elevated cortisol levels.[5] The Framingham Heart Study revealed that people with the highest cortisol performed worse on memory and attention tests while showing brain changes typical of Alzheimer's precursors. The hippocampus (memory area) of your brain shrinks.[6]

A research paper that reviewed and analyzed data from multiple studies of more than 3,000 participants found significant cardiovascular responses during rumination, with particularly damaging effects on blood pressure. All age groups showed that rumination compromises immune function—affecting white blood cell counts and natural killer cell activity—while activating inflammatory pathways contributing to cardiovascular disease and other chronic conditions.[7]

Thought suppression also affects behavior. Dr. James Erskine is a senior lecturer in psychology and behavioral medicine at City St George's, University of London. His research interests include intrusive thoughts, thought suppression, repressive coping, aging, leadership and health outcomes, resilience, counseling psychology, and existential psychotherapy. His controlled experiments revealed that people who suppressed thoughts about chocolate subsequently ate more chocolate than the control groups. Smokers who suppressed smoking thoughts showed an initial reduction during suppression, but significantly increased smoking afterward. Craving for opioids likewise increases.[8] Suppression doesn't eliminate desires—it amplifies them, leading to the behaviors people are trying to avoid.

Treatment Approaches Must Change

Despite the overwhelming evidence that thought suppression is harmful, most therapeutic approaches still focus on managing or controlling thoughts rather than addressing the underlying threat physiology that drives both the thoughts and thwarts suppression attempts. The mainstream contemporary approaches to mental health—based on thought modification—are inherently flawed. Rather than trying to manage thoughts directly, people must learn thought separation techniques to help neutralize the physiological threat states that drive them.

There are many ways to achieve separation from your thoughts. Remember, thoughts are not the problem; it is your reaction to them that creates physiological changes and internal chaos. Writing allows you to observe them and suspend judgment. The visual, tactile experience of physically writing your thoughts on paper and discarding them creates space between you and your thoughts. This works on both a conscious and unconscious level.

Expressive Writing

Dr. James W. Pennebaker, Professor Emeritus of Psychology at the University of Texas at Austin, conceptualized expressive writing and began publishing on it in 1986.[9] His initial research involved college student volunteers who were asked to write for fifteen minutes a day, for four consecutive days. There were four groups:

1. The control group wrote about trivial topics.
2. The trauma-emotion group wrote about feelings about a traumatic event.
3. The trauma-fact group wrote only facts about the event.
4. The trauma-emotion-fact group wrote about the whole experience.

The groups that included emotional details in their writing had the most health benefits and ended up visiting the student health center over the next six months at about half the rate that students in the control group did. The participants in the trauma-emotion and trauma-emotion-fact groups experienced initial physiological arousal when first writing and reliving their traumas, and also experienced long-term decreases in their overall health problems.

The proven benefits of expressive writing are numerous. Improvements have been noted across multiple domains, including physical, mental, immune function, performance, and disease states. Here is a short list of the benefits of expressive writing:

- improved sleep
- better academic performance
- optimized athletic performance
- decreased pain
- improved energy and less fatigue
- reduced symptoms in autoimmune disorders, including:
    - rheumatoid arthritis
    - systemic lupus erythematosus
    - ankylosing spondylitis

    - multiple sclerosis
    - inflammatory bowel disease
- fewer irritable bowel symptoms
- better function in patients with fibromyalgia
- improved breathing in moderately severe asthma patients
- decreased viral load in HIV patients and improved survival
- lower blood pressure
- reduced symptoms of depression
- less reactivity in PTSD
- smoking cessation
- improved working memory
- breaking through writer's block
- improved problem solving
- better sleep

For a more exhaustive review, please refer to *Opening Up by Writing It Down* by Dr. Pennebaker and Dr. Joshua M. Smyth, two pioneers in this field of research.[10] Further research is needed to determine the most effective methods of expressive writing for individuals in light of their specific medical concerns and backgrounds. The bottom line is that some form of expressive writing enhances both our physical and mental health.

In an elegant essay, "The Seed of Our Undoing," Dr. Daniel Wegner noted that the need for mental control was a powerful force in driving ruminations.[11] He felt there were few answers, but the one strategy that decreased their impact was to write down the thoughts and express the emotions being suppressed. The deeper the emotional expression, the better. He observed that some people would occasionally decompensate, and the exercise needed to be done under psychological supervision. This is consistent with Dr. Pennebaker's observation that more intense emotional expression was activating. Expressive writing can connect you to some disturbing memories.

The Practice

Based on this observation that deep emotional expression can be disruptive, I recommend that you write your stream of consciousness at a manageable level. If it feels destabilizing, either stop or lower the intensity of your expression. Then, as soon as you've completed your writing session, destroy your pages. Tear them into small pieces and dispose of them. Some people prefer to shred or burn them. The important thing is that you write with absolute freedom.

This is simply a separation exercise—no more and no less. Many issues might seem to arise during it, but they are just thoughts. Do not pause to analyze them, as this will only reinforce their presence. Write and then discard. Do this for a few minutes once or twice a day. Make it a habit, like brushing your teeth. Even when your RUTs or pain lessens, continue expressive writing as a daily practice to maintain your well-being. You might feel frustrated because you don't know what to write or because the same thoughts keep recurring. That's okay. If this happens, one alternative approach is to doodle on a piece of paper. If a word comes to mind, jot it down and continue doodling. You don't have to dig for unwanted thoughts; they emerge in their own time.

The duration and time of day don't matter. You are the one in charge. You can write for as little as thirty seconds or for hours. Some people write once or twice a day, either in the morning or before bedtime, or both. The main issue is making it a habit that fits into your life. Remember, this process should not feel like work. Separation exercises are the first step in reprogramming your brain.

Mechanical Meditation (The Freight Train)

As pointed out in chapter 4, your brain is constantly changing and adapting to sensory input. You can reprogram it in any way you wish. There are three components of the programming process that stimulate neuroplastic changes in your brain: awareness, separation, and reprogramming. Expressive writing combines awareness and separation into a single exercise. Reprogramming is a separate but linked process that we will get to in chapter 10. With expressive writing, it is important to separate from *all* your thoughts, both negative and positive. Through cognitive fusion, your identity is also connected to positive self-narratives. Changing your brain involves connecting to the moment you are in, as opposed to reacting to some event in the past, pleasant or not.

Imagine a long, fully loaded freight train. Remarkably powerful engines have been designed to pull such a heavy load, even up a steep incline. This is not so different from how we carry our past into the present, and still function. However, at some tipping point, we may reach our limit. Expressive writing almost instantly disconnects you from the past. It fosters an awareness of what lives in the train cars of your life. The space generated between you and the thoughts that are now on paper create a physical sense of separation. It is not entirely clear why this works, but the exercise requires a conscious act on your part, while the sensations of sight and feel are unconsciously processed by your nervous system. You are making the thoughts "real" and then distancing yourself. It's as if you have unhooked the first car from the engine. Skilled meditators can attain thought separation through visualization, but expressive writing is an excellent initial, concrete step. You can consider it mechanical meditation.

No rule of life says you must stay connected to such a huge load of freight. Disconnect from each train car until your engine is pulling nothing. Now you are better able to fully engage in the present moment. Think of all that energy you have freed up to direct toward more enjoyable, creative pursuits. You can spend a lifetime trying to unload the freight or take a few minutes to disconnect from all the cars and leave your past behind.

Verbal Expression

Verbalizing your thoughts (simply hearing them) is another strategy for externalizing them. The separation is occurring through an auditory route instead of through sight and feel. In his book *Feeling Good*, Dr. David Burns recommends standing in front of a mirror and conversing with the person reflected in it, using the self-critical voice in your head.[12] Naturally, with nobody else around, you can express yourself without restraint. You would never talk to anyone else in that manner, would you?

I must admit, when I was struggling with RUTs and tried it for the first time, it was unsettling, but effective. Talking to my reflection in the mirror caused a significant shift in my perspective: I quickly recognized the irrationality and toxicity of these thoughts. You can also simply speak aloud to yourself, without a mirror. You can use this strategy whenever you need a reality check. Just don't try this verbal approach while you are driving; I learned this the hard way, with several close calls in downtown Seattle!

Switch to the Third Person

One research paper examined the effect of verbally switching negative self-talk from the first person to the third person. Using functional MRI scans, the research team observed people using both approaches. They showed this third-person approach calmed the amygdala region (known as the danger signal area) without activating the higher cognitive functions of the brain. Verbalizing negative self-talk in the third person bypassed the need to use mental strategies to manage anxiety.[13]

Alternative "Writing" Approaches

Some patients have told me that when they wake up in the middle of the night, they "write" their RUTs in the air or on the palm of their hand. One gentleman wrote on his chest with one finger. A woman kept a pad of paper next to her at night and would scribble on it in the dark. After doing this, she could usually fall back asleep quickly. A physician friend of mine envisioned himself sitting in a theater, watching himself perform scenes from different roles he has played throughout his life. This helped him to create a sense of separation between his past and the present. He pictured both negative and positive experiences, creating space to change direction in the present instead of automatically reacting.

If you become frustrated because you don't know what to write or because the same thoughts keep recurring, that's perfectly normal and okay. Get creative and try a different approach. Again, it can be helpful to doodle until more words spring to mind.

Background Observations

When I began exploring the data on expressive writing, I was amazed to discover that over 1,400 studies in the literature show its healing power for both mental and physical disorders. When I spoke with Dr. Smyth, he confirmed my clinical observations. I couldn't believe medical schools didn't routinely teach this well-documented healing strategy. They still don't.

When our informal scientific discussion group spoke with Dr. Pennebaker, we asked him why he believed this method has such wide-ranging beneficial effects. He observed that it's a nonthreatening way to release secrets. We all have parts of our past and ourselves that we are not proud of, and it takes significant metabolic and cognitive energy to keep them hidden. With this exercise, you don't need to confess or speak to anyone; you write your thoughts, allowing yourself to separate from them. This is very different than suppressing or fighting them. Dr. Pennebaker also believes that seeing your thoughts allows you to reshape the narrative of your life. He emphasizes that expressive writing is not a catharsis; you are not dumping or getting rid of your thoughts and frustrations. They might well come back again at another time. It is simply an exercise to help you separate from them and reconnect to the present, allowing space for other thoughts to enter your mind.

Resistance

While I was coming out of my abyss of chronic pain, expressive writing was a critical starting point. In 2000, intuition told me that my patients would benefit from it. Indeed, patients who tried expressive writing improved, but I frequently encountered significant resistance from others. The patients who would not engage in this simple exercise did not have good outcomes. I eventually learned that the extent of a patient's resistance was an indicator of whether we could work together. Here are my observations of why people resist:

Expressive writing seems too simple. You might wonder how it could have such a profound impact on such a huge problem, yet its effectiveness is well documented.

Expressive writing requires letting go of the illusion of control. Letting go of your control strategies can be disconcerting and challenging. Expressive writing is a defined action that moves you forward in the face of this deep resistance and helps you break through.

You might feel that your suffering is not being adequately acknowledged. "Are you kidding me? How is this addressing my years of intense pain and suffering?" You might feel dismissed and insulted when your doctor recommends expressive writing. Don't. Research shows that the impact of chronic pain on the quality of your life is comparable to having terminal cancer. I understand the gravity of your suffering. However, I have seen both personally and professionally how powerful this exercise can be as a healing strategy, alongside others.

Your anxiety might initially increase. Since cognitive fusion causes you to feel you are your thoughts, separating from them can feel threatening. When you begin expressive writing, your anxiety might initially increase, causing the opposite effect of what you wanted or expected. As long as it's not too intense, it is important to keep moving through this initial discomfort.

A professor once came to me for a surgical consultation regarding spinal stenosis in his lower back, which is the narrowing of the spinal canal. This condition was exerting pressure on his nerves and causing significant leg pain. I believed he would benefit from a straightforward procedure called a laminotomy to relieve the pressure. Following my protocol of rehabbing patients before surgery, I suggested he practice expressive writing for a few weeks before we made a final decision. He hesitated. I insisted I wouldn't perform his surgery without his first making this simple effort toward his recovery. He returned a few weeks later and laughed, saying, "This is ridiculous. I started writing, and my pain was gone within a week!" He began implementing the rest of my recommendations; years later, he remains pain-free. While he might need surgery someday, why subject him to the risks of back surgery when he feels fine today?

Years earlier, when I first gave expressive writing a try, I had no idea it would alleviate my prolonged suffering. Yet, after two weeks of writing, I noticed a definite shift in my mood; and six weeks later, I began to feel much better. This occurred after I had been struggling with RUTs and other mental and physical pain symptoms for fifteen years. Expressive writing has been a part of my life ever since. All I have to do is stop for a few weeks, and I am reminded of its power. Two or three of my symptoms will reappear and quickly resolve when I reengage.

However, don't use the professor's story or mine as the norm. Most people experience a subtle but noticeable shift in a few weeks or months. Do not get discouraged, even if prolonged efforts appear to have no impact. Expressive writing is rarely a definitive solution by itself. Rather, it is one small but vital step in your healing journey. I have seen few people heal without regularly using it as a foundation for the rest of their healing process. Expressive writing is a tool to be used indefinitely, at a level that is comfortable.

Let's consider another foundational anchoring and calming practice: active meditation. I highly recommend active meditation alongside expressive writing as two complementary healing practices.

Active Meditation

You cannot fix, repair, or outrun RUTs, but one option is to shift your focus away from them and activate more functional, enjoyable circuits. Focusing your attention on a specific sensation from your immediate surroundings quickly accomplishes this. Using any type of sensory input—sound, smell, taste, feel, touch, sight—works. My term for this tool is *active meditation*—essentially an abbreviated version of a mindfulness meditation. Focus on any one sensation from your immediate surroundings for a few seconds, or up to a minute. Then you can shift to other sensations, but focus on one at a time. This connects your consciousness to the present. Incorporate this practice frequently into your daily routine until it becomes habitual.

I first learned about this type of sensory meditation at a meditation retreat given by Alan Wallace, a prominent researcher in integrating Buddhist contemplative practices with Western science. He emphasized three interconnected steps from his mindfulness practice based on Tibetan Buddhism: relaxation, stabilization, and sensation. His meditation lasted for a few minutes, but as I incorporated it into my surgical practice, I learned it was also effective when done frequently for as little as five to ten seconds at a time.[14]

Active Meditation on the Run

Active meditation is a remarkably effective practice for staying calm throughout the day. Whatever I am doing, I will focus on the most relevant sensation. Eating is relaxing, but even more so when you actually focus on how the food tastes. When I was a little wound up during clinic, I would engage in active meditation with my patients. Here were the basic steps:

1. Sit back in our chairs, letting our shoulders sag and jaws relax.
2. Take a deep breath and let it go (relaxation).
3. Stay in this state for five to ten seconds (stabilization).

4. Sequentially focus on the most available sensory input, one sense at a time (sensation).

For example, the sound of the ventilation system was an easy starting point. Then we would shift our attention to people's voices outside the door, then to feeling our feet on the floor, and back to the vent. It only took about a minute. Invariably, everyone in the room would feel more relaxed. I could hear that my voice had changed to a lower pitch. We had shifted our attention from our racing thoughts to the current moment through sensory awareness. It is an exercise that I encouraged them to do often, until it became automatic.

We also practiced active meditation in the operating room, each of us using our instruments with a light touch. Eventually, it became automatic. Surgery transformed from being an intense experience into a graceful team effort—where we connected with every move and sensation and communicated well. There was a significant drop in technical complications and an increase in enjoyment during surgery. The benefits of this sensory approach also carried over into our daily lives.

At any point in the day, pausing for as little as three to five seconds to focus on a single sensation can help to separate you from your thoughts and calm your nervous system.

Deep Listening

Another method of thought separation is deep listening—that is, listening in a way that allows you to visualize the other person's perspective and realize that the words they are saying to you have a different meaning to them than they do to you. It is remarkable how much more interesting the world is when you quit continually trying to impose your perspective on it.

I focused on family dynamics for the last few years of my clinical practice. Family members are powerful triggers that keep people stuck. I have found very few exceptions to this rule. I would challenge my patients to practice deep listening while offering no advice or criticism to any family member for a month. None. Many medical professionals, including myself, have placed this approach into the realm of "soft science" and dismissed it. That is not true. Nonthreatening sensory input calms your nervous system and lowers threat physiology. This is not a psychological exercise.

Summary

One of the most powerful ways to stimulate and reinforce RUTs is to suppress unpleasant emotions. Inadvertently, the ongoing battle deeply embeds them in your nervous system. This interaction causes cognitive fusion, where your identity becomes entangled with your thoughts. The tragedy is that our identity is negatively biased because 90 percent of our thoughts reflect our body's ongoing surveillance for threat.

Being nonreactive to your thoughts is a way of separating from your thoughts. This is in contrast with analyzing, fighting, rationalizing, or suppressing them, which gives them a lot of power. Two basic and effective approaches are expressive writing and active meditation. Expressive writing involves writing your thoughts on paper in a stream of consciousness. Knowing that you will immediately destroy the paper rather than analyze what you've written allows you to express your thoughts and emotions freely. Active meditation is the practice of shifting your focus from unwanted thoughts to another sensation and holding that focus for anywhere from a few seconds for up to a few minutes. The goal is to do it as frequently as possible, so it becomes automatic. By crowding out RUTs with other sensory inputs, you can keep connecting to the present moment.

In the framework of Dynamic Healing, both strategies change the nature of your sensory input. By choosing more functional and pleasant input, you'll indirectly lower your threat physiology toward safety. By reconnecting to the present moment, you are bringing your brain back online. With increased awareness that you are not your thoughts, you gain perspective and create space for new sensations.

In the next chapter, we will discuss the role of threat physiology in driving RUTs, and how RUTs simultaneously cause threat physiology. It is a bidirectional feedback loop. But negative thoughts are not the only inputs causing you stress. Since there are many other inputs feeding your threat physiology, calming down your stress response requires a separate skill set. Stop energizing your RUTs. Learning how to calm your physiology will free up energy to connect with the present and enjoy your life.

CHAPTER 8

Calm Your Physiology

Nothing can bring you peace but yourself.
—RALPH WALDO EMERSON, *Essays: First Series*

We have all, at one point or another, been blindsided by our threat physiology. Some of us struggle with this more than others, and sometimes we spend our whole lives in this state. I have had the professional privilege of witnessing hundreds of people heal from chronic pain through Dynamic Healing. The exact method of calming the nervous system doesn't matter, but I've observed that the tipping point is *always* in addressing anger. Minor improvements in RUTs and mental states can occur using different tools, but deep, transformative healing won't happen while you are in a constant state of fight-or-flight.

So much of calming our physiology hinges on anger. Anger is temporary insanity. It is a deadly loop that builds on itself. I did not realize I was angry until I was fifty years old. How is that possible? Since adolescence, my self-image had been one of toughness. I refused to let anything bother me. My nickname in high school and college was "the brick." "Bring it on. You can't hurt me" was my attitude.

At age thirty-seven, and only four years into my practice, I broke down. During my subsequent thirteen years of psychotherapy, my symptoms worsened dramatically, especially the RUTs. I still did not have a clue that I might be angry. In fact, in 2001, on my first date with my future wife, I told her I had ADD and OCD, but I had worked through my anger issues. To this day, I don't understand why Babs stuck with me. I thought I had worked on them; I had discussed anger many times with my therapists, gone to workshops, and read many self-help books. Intellectually, I knew a lot about anger, but I had built up a façade of being enlightened. I became more attached to my created identity than to discovering who I actually was. I was a cauldron of repressed anger.

You would think that falling in love would improve things, but over the next year, my condition deteriorated. It wasn't until Mother's Day 2002 that the word *victim* flickered in my mind. I was in Oakland, California, spending the weekend with my future wife, Babs. She and her daughter were washing the car on a beautiful day. I vividly recall standing on the front porch watching them and thinking that life could not get better than this, yet I was miserable. I don't know why the word *victim* crossed my mind. It was a label that I had never applied to myself. I disliked the word and was critical of those who seemed to play that role. Over the next twelve months, all hell broke loose, which was even more intense than my experience in 1990, when all of this began with that panic attack on a bridge. Suddenly, I was exposed to my lifetime of repressed anger with no knowledge of how to deal with it. I became incredibly emotionally unstable, and I continued to be amazed that Babs was sticking with me.

I read any book or article on anger that I could find. David Burns's *Feeling Good* was especially impactful.[1] He said to write, so I wrote—a lot. I wrote following his three-column technique, which we will revisit in chapter 9. In the first column, I wrote down what I now recognize as cognitive distortions. In the second column, I placed these thoughts in one of the ten categories Burns describes. Then I wrote a more rational thought in the third column. At the time, I did not know the term *expressive writing* and its various applications. Within a few weeks of acknowledging my victim role, I felt a shift, and I dove in more deeply, spending hours writing. It was an intense experience to realize that most of my thoughts and emotions were based on cognitive distortions. I felt some relief, but at the same time, the process of stripping away my identity put me into a free fall. I felt intense, raw emotions that I had not known I was capable of, both highs and lows. The swings would occur quickly, and I no longer had the protection of my rigid identity.

After six months of struggling, I gave up the battle. It felt like I was in a silent chamber, with nowhere to turn. I felt peaceful, and my mind quieted down. Over the next few months, my physical and mental symptoms began to resolve; and a year later, all of them were gone. Over twenty years later, I am continuing to deepen my understanding of the healing process—how it was possible for me to heal and thrive.

This is not the way to address anger. I took a long, torturous road. At the time, I had no awareness of the power of threat physiology, and no strategies to calm myself. I gave up fighting only because my reserves were depleted. Since then, I have watched hundreds of people heal by recognizing their anger (and victimhood) and using effective strategies to process it. Anger is a universal experience, and it manifests in various ways. You don't have to wait for the top to blow off the pressure cooker before you address it.

Data shows that over 80 percent of people suffering from chronic pain have not forgiven the person or situation that hurt them.[2] Ultimately, the person they are the most furious at is themselves. Dr. John E. Sarno, a famous rehab doctor and author of several best-selling books, called this sensation "rage."[3] When you are carrying repressed rage, you aren't aware of the depth and breadth of your anger, yet your threat physiology is destroying your body from the inside out. Why wouldn't you become ill?

Anger is a meta-problem, meaning this physiological state blocks the higher thinking needed to understand that you are angry. It is hard to solve a problem that you don't know exists, much less understand in detail. Finding a creative solution to any challenge requires awareness of the particulars. People typically focus on symptoms without addressing the deeper problem and driving force of the anger. But how do we cut through the symptoms (manifestations of anger) to create space for our anger so we can recognize it, separate from it, and calm our physiology? It might help to begin by conceptualizing a sequence of healing, using the metaphor of a tree.

The C-quence of Healing

We can think of the sequential steps to healing as connection, confidence, and creativity—or what I call the C-quence of healing. It promotes a shift from a reactive to a creative state. The roots, trunk, and branches of a tree correspond to each of the three Cs.

The Roots of Connection

Think of yourself as a tree, and the past as the ground beneath you. Every moment of your life experience serves as a foundation for your current

"Neuroshment"

I want to introduce you to Rita, who came to me as a patient in 2014 and holds the record in my practice for enduring pain the longest before finding relief. She suffered for fifty-five years and was still able to heal at age seventy-eight.

Rita had experienced severe anxiety, migratory body pain, and mood swings for over fifty years. She had explored every avenue in the medical system without success. The first year of working with her was challenging. She collaborated with one of my pain colleagues, applying the approaches presented in this book. We were not optimistic about her prognosis, as her progress was so erratic.

Over the course of a year, she broke free of her pain symptoms and remained that way for over ten years before passing away. Like everyone else, she faced significant setbacks that caused her pain to flare. Much of it was mental pain, but she learned to cope, understand her triggers, navigate through the dark spots, and move on.

Babs and I knew her well and discovered that she possessed a remarkable depth of wisdom and creativity. She was an eager learner with an impressive grasp of awareness, choice, and neuroplasticity. One comment that caught our attention was a word she coined: "neuroshment." The tree metaphor originated with this word. According to this remarkable woman, the main question we need to ask ourselves is, "What can I learn to help me live my life better today? What will 'neurosh' my brain for growth and change?" We must dig deeper with our roots and reach higher with our branches.

actions, learning, and growth. The more expansive and versatile your root system, the greater your chances of surviving and thriving. The concept that "you have to feel to heal" has existed for many centuries. Engaging intentionally with the painful emotions under the ground is fundamental to the healing process.

In order to separate from your thoughts, you must become aware of their content. This is especially true in light of the phenomenon of cognitive fusion, where you are so intertwined with your thoughts that they have become your identity. Every unpleasant memory feels like a part of you today, so you instinctively fight them to defend yourself. These memories have effectively become you. The roots represent the nervous system connecting you to all of your memories, conscious and unconscious, and the feelings associated with each one. Unfortunately, if you had an angry and chaotic past, these memories and associated feelings probably dominate your nervous system. If you have spent years suppressing them under hard, compacted soil, you have compromised your root system and its ability to absorb nutrients. As you break up the mental rigidity and loosen the soil, you'll create the space you need to learn from the old programming and branch out your root system.

When you suppress thoughts and emotions, you block conscious connection to your past while still unconsciously reacting to it. I am continually challenged to help people understand what is blocking their healing. People often fail to let go of how they were mistreated as children, which is the most common scenario I have encountered. The best intervention in these cases is to introduce them to calming tools or suggest they see a therapist to get their thinking brain back online. Then I invite them back when they feel ready to move forward.

If the soil of your past is hard and dry, your root system will develop poorly and fail to absorb nutrients. Softening the soil allows the root system to develop into an intricate network. Preparing the soil is an ongoing, deliberate choice—and for most of us, it means processing our anger. The first step is to recognize anger when it occurs. As discussed in chapter 3, there is a sequence to anger: (1) real or perceived unpleasant circumstance, (2) blame, (3) victimhood, (4) anger. Few of us want to admit to playing the victim role, so we disguise it. It is also potent and addictive, so unconsciously, we don't want to let go of it. Here are a few of the common disguises to victimhood and anger:

- needing to be "right"
- feeling frustrated
- feeling sorry for yourself
- being in denial
- disassociating—closing the door on the past
- rationalizing that you are not really angry
- constantly people-pleasing
- adhering to a "cool and calm" identity
- judging and labeling
- holding yourself and others to high ideals and standards
- being perfectionistic
- being opinionated

These behaviors don't always indicate that you're suppressing anger, but they are often instinctively used to disguise it. Consider your own victim disguises. Be honest with yourself and write them down. Don't throw this list away. Occasionally look at it to remind yourself to notice how you keep playing out these deeply embedded patterns. As you nurture awareness, you'll be amazed at how often you play the victim.

There is a common perception that adversity is necessary for personal growth. This can be true, to a point, but I would add that most people grow best when they experience adversity within a context of safety and support—not in environments of relentless threat or deprivation. Recent research suggests that adversity does not precipitate growth in the vast majority of people.[4] Therefore, open up yourself to your past safely and gradually. It can take time to reconnect with your roots in a constructive way. Connecting with others is also essential. A healthy, mature tree not only has deep roots but also connects with the root systems of other trees for nutrient exchange and stability.

The Trunk of Confidence

Confidence grows as you learn to engage with a wide range of thoughts and emotions at face value, without the interventions of an ego based on cognitive distortions. As you learn how to separate your thoughts from your ego, you will become less reactive. Lowering your physiology from threat to safety dampens reactivity. In chapter 9, we will explore the relationship between the ego and mental rigidity, and how to soften them to enhance awareness and neuroplasticity. As you develop cognitive flexibility, you will be able to rise to any challenge. Similar to the expanding trunk of a tree, your self-confidence will grow.

The Branches of Creativity

There is a limit to how much you can benefit from ongoing personal work. You end up stirring the same pot. Deep healing occurs when you expand your conscious awareness upward and outward, like branches reaching for the sun. This is how you stimulate new circuitry in your brain. These new circuits form apart from your embedded pain circuits, allowing you to create more functional and enjoyable experiences. Creative engagement is the definitive answer for RUTs and pain. Once you are firmly grounded in your reality, you will be amazed at how far and freely your branches can grow. We will discuss creativity in chapter 10.

Directly Lower Threat Physiology (Output)

In the Dynamic Healing framework, the output is the state of your physiology. Your nervous system collects a massive amount of incoming data every second and assimilates it all. The nervous system analyzes the data to determine if it is safe or threatening and then sends signals. The input, the nervous system, and the output are in a complex, dynamic relationship, and this is why it's ineffective to address only one variable at a time. It is critical to remember that *anxiety* and *anger* are words that describe these survival sensations. They are not who you are. Visualization is a powerful strategy for depersonalizing them.

Picture a large thermometer on a wall that reflects the level of your stress chemicals. Use the term *elevated stress chemicals* instead of *anxiety* or *anger*. Then, use any of the following calming activities to lower the temperature. "Watching" it go up or down provides feedback about the effectiveness of your approach.

In chapter 7, we talked about expressive writing as a necessary tool for creating thought separation, and for many people it's an effective first step. However, if you find that it initially over-activates you, causing you to feel emotionally unstable or exacerbating a mental health issue, begin with these calming strategies. Learn a few of them well, as you'll be using them indefinitely. Spend as much time as you need until you feel some of the calming effects. Understanding the nature of RUTs by revisiting the concepts we've covered in this book and continuing to learn from related resources is also important. Knowledge provides a sense of control, which stimulates the production of anti-inflammatory cytokines.

Several activities decrease anxiety and anger by activating the anti-inflammatory effects of the vagus nerve, the tenth cranial nerve. Each of these strategies stimulates a nerve near the vagus origin in the midbrain.

Calming Activities

Bear with me for a moment as we briefly delve into the key players in the nervous system that make calming activities so effective. There are twelve cranial nerves that originate in the midbrain, just above the spinal cord. Cranial nerves originate directly from the brain, as opposed to spinal nerves that branch off from the spinal cord. The origins of these nerves are groups of neurons called nuclei. They contain the cell bodies of that specific nerve.

The vagus nerve, the tenth cranial nerve, is the core of the calming PNS. The nuclei close to the vagus nucleus include the fifth, seventh, and eighth cranial nerves. The fifth is the trigeminal nerve that has three major divisions, with one covering the forehead. The seventh supplies part of the face and the back of the throat, and the eighth innervates the auditory nerve. Stimulating any of these nerves affects the tenth cranial vagus nerve. Now let's briefly take a closer look at each.

Fifth Cranial Nerve: Forehead

You have probably seen someone lie down with a cold pack on their forehead, or perhaps you have done it yourself. Or you've instinctively massaged your forehead in a moment of stress. These are effective tools for stimulating the fifth cranial trigeminal nerve. Use them as often as you can. Don't wait for a crisis.

Seventh Cranial Nerve: Humming and Singing

The seventh cranial facial nerve innervates the muscles of the throat and back of your tongue. Humming and singing activate this nerve, which is close to the vagus nucleus. Many people find it to be an easy, enjoyable, quick way to relax. Try it and consider making it a regular habit.

Eighth Cranial Nerve: Auditory

The auditory route stimulates the eighth cranial nerve and is a powerful way to calm down. Here are some ways to stimulate the eight cranial nerve:

- Listen to soft music, such as lullabies or soothing classical music.
- Listen to any music that you find relaxing. Try music that takes you back to a time in your life when you were full of joy and hope.
- Use various auditory therapies designed to stimulate the eighth cranial nerve. For example, Dr. Stephen Porges and his team developed an approach called the Safe and Sound Protocol. They administer it through earphones, filtering out threatening tones of lower pitch.
- See an auricular (ear) acupuncturist who can apply small acupuncture needles at specific points on the earlobe to stimulate the nerve.

A member of my coaching group, a woman from England, had just begun her healing journey. Struggling with severe RUTs and burning sensations all over her body, she had an experience that she feared I would consider "loony." While babysitting her baby granddaughter, her RUTs and pain were worse than usual, and she couldn't wait to leave. She played a lullaby to calm her granddaughter, and noticed her own pain was gone for the first time in many months. She was concerned that this was all psychological. I explained to her it was a clear example of the calming, anti-inflammatory power of the vagus nerve, and she had stimulated it through the auditory route. Making this kind of connection is a major step forward in the healing process.

Breathing Exercises

Breathing exercises directly stimulate the vagus nerve, and there are many options to choose from. Find a few that you enjoy and implement them throughout your day.

- Practice slow breathing at a rate of six to ten breaths per minute. Breathe in and out slowly for about five minutes. (It is not necessary to pay constant attention to your breath, as this is not a meditative technique.)
- Take a deep breath in and then breathe out as slowly as you can through pursed lips. Whenever you feel stressed during the day, do

this quick exercise. Do this four to five times a day, for a minute or two, as needed.

- Breathe through your nose to stimulate the release of nitric oxide. About 90 percent of people normally breathe through their noses, but when stress activates the sympathetic nervous system, breathing becomes rapid and shallow, frequently leading to mouth breathing and potentially increasing anxiety. Chronic stress can lead to habitual mouth breathing. Here is a suggested approach:

    1. Sit or stand in a relaxed position, shoulders down.
    2. Close your mouth and inhale gently through your nose, allowing your belly—not your chest—to expand.
    3. Exhale gently and completely through your nose, feeling your abdomen fall.
    4. Continue this slow, even breathing for several minutes, focusing on the sensation of air moving in and out of your nostrils. To help slow your breath, you can try inhaling for a count of four, and exhaling for a count of six (counting silently).

- Breathe through alternate nostrils. Here is one approach:

    1. Sit comfortably with a straight spine.
    2. Place your left hand on your knee. With your right hand, use your thumb to close your right nostril.
    3. Inhale slowly through your left nostril.
    4. Close your left nostril with your right ring finger, release your thumb, and exhale through your right nostril.
    5. Inhale through your right nostril.
    6. Close your right nostril with your thumb, release your ring finger, and exhale through your left nostril.
    7. This completes one full cycle. Continue for three to five cycles, or for several minutes as is comfortable. Always keep the breath smooth and steady; never force it.

Direct Vagal Nerve Stimulation

Direct Vagal Nerve Stimulation (VNS) increases serotonin and dopamine, reduces inflammation, and supports neural plasticity—all changes that have been linked with improved mood and reduced repetitive negative thinking. Here are some data points to consider:

- A study on chronic worriers found that transcutaneous VNS (tVNS) reduced spontaneous negative thought intrusions, with participants reporting fewer unwanted recurrent worries during stimulation.[5]
- VNS successfully helps patients manage obsessive thinking and emotional distress by lowering hyperactivity in the amygdala and PFC, treating treatment-resistant OCD. Clinical trials found VNS improved mood, reduced anxiety, and decreased compulsive symptoms.[6]
- VNS is consistently shown to improve autonomic regulation, reduce physiological reactivity (lower cortisol, improve heart rate variability), and enhance emotional regulation in stress-related psychiatric conditions, including PTSD and depression—contexts where rumination is problematic.[7]

These direct approaches are accessible through many providers who are familiar with calming approaches to regulating a dysregulated autonomic nervous system. You can look up "vagal nerve stimulation," "Safe and Sound Protocol,"[8] or HRV biofeedback. Direct VNS is becoming increasingly available.[9] It is not a solution by itself but can be a useful adjunct to your overall care. Consider it in the context of your whole-body healing plan.

The State of Your Nervous System

In the Dynamic Healing framework, your nervous system is a complex relay system. Every response reflects the quality of input from the various external and internal sensors and also the state of your nervous system. You can be hypersensitive, requiring less intense input to create a threat response; or calm, requiring more intense input to elicit a response. Anti-inflammatory strategies create a more stable and resilient nervous system. The four most foundational ones address sleep, diet, exercise, and fostering a safe relationship with your past with a skilled professional. While it's common knowledge that improved sleep, nutrition, physical fitness, and self-awareness are important to overall well-being, we don't always consider these factors in light of threat versus safety physiology.

Sleep

Adequate sleep is a top priority, and a prerequisite for physiological healing. During my years of surgical practice, I always asked new patients if they were getting enough sleep, and would not move forward with treatment until I was satisfied they were getting regular rest. Usually within six weeks, we had a reasonable handle on it. Sometimes patients needed medication for a few months to help them transition to a better sleep pattern. As the nervous system calmed down, we could minimize the meds quickly.

Research shows that a lack of sleep causes chronic lower back pain, and not the other way around.[10] A single night of poor sleep can increase pain by approximately 50 percent the following day.[11] The same is true for the frequency of RUTs. One paper demonstrated that one night of poor sleep increased repetitive unwanted thoughts by 50 percent, and they persisted for a few weeks after the study.[12]

If you are still struggling to get enough sleep, make it the highest priority to resolve this issue. Many resources are available, including chapter 14 of my book *Back in Control.*

Diet

If you immediately associate the word *diet* with weight loss, forget about weight loss for now. When you're feeling better, you might want to pursue it, but when you're struggling with anxiety and RUTs, you don't need the added stress. Most of us could or should lose weight, yet few of us actually do. Why? One reason is that the body is remarkably efficient at retaining calories. The other, more important reason is that when we are overwhelmed by life, including RUTs, we don't have the mental energy to pursue a diet. Besides, emotional eating works—it floods your brain with wonderful sensory input.

A more constructive goal to consider is to adopt an anti-inflammatory diet. There are many excellent books on the topic, along with simple, effective methods to incorporate more anti-inflammatory foods into your diet. However, it is essential to stay flexible with yourself and focus on long-term behavioral changes rather than rigidly adhering to rules.

As a surgeon, I am not a diet expert. Surgeons often have some of the worst eating habits I know, myself included. We are so busy that the time we take to eat feels like a waste or delays us from getting home. I sat down to lunch one day with a fellow of mine, who was consuming two large Pepsis and three bags of popcorn. Many surgeons eat better, but everyone is in a hurry. My wake-up call came during a routine physical when I found my liver functions were sky-high. I am not a drinker, and it didn't make sense. It turns out that sugar can be deadly. For example, when people develop cirrhosis of the liver, it's the sugar causing inflammation that leads to damage, not necessarily alcohol.[13] At that point in my career, I would eat an entire package of Oreo cookies without a second thought. Talk about emotional eating. I quickly cut down on my sugar intake, and six months later, my liver functions returned to normal.

One way to lower inflammatory markers is through time-restricted eating within an eight- to twelve-hour window. It's not very hard to do, and it quickly becomes a routine. There are also various intermittent fasting regimes you might consider.[14]

I am not a fan of strict diets, as they are rarely sustainable. I believe having a basic understanding of nutrition helps you make smarter choices. A friend of mine, Dr. Rob Lustig, lives just a few miles from me and works at the University of California, San Francisco. He is a well-known pediatric endocrinologist and neuroendocrinologist, recognized for his research and public education on childhood obesity, sugar metabolism, and metabolic health. In his book *Fat Chance: Beating the Odds Against Sugar, Processed Food, Obesity, and Disease,* he explains the biochemistry of food in a straightforward way, helping people make better decisions.[15] It's no coincidence that 60 percent of Americans are worried about their weight. Ten large multinational companies control the world's food supply and must heavily process it to keep it from spoiling. It is a serious public health problem, often hidden.

Another accessible book on the principles of healthy eating is *The Forks Over Knives Plan* by wife-and-husband team Dr. Alona Pulde and Dr. Matt Lederman and three other contributors.[16] She is a family practitioner and developed the lifestyle change program used for patients in the *Forks Over Knives* documentary. He is an internist and also appeared in the film. Along with other doctors and researchers behind the film, they assert that "modern diseases can be prevented and often reversed by leaving meat, dairy, and highly refined foods off the plate and adopting a whole-food, plant-based diet instead." Dr. Pulde and Dr. Lederman are also friends of mine, and they have significantly influenced my views on diet and nutrition.

The effects of ultra-processed foods have been found to include chronic elevations of inflammatory markers, increased incidence of all chronic inflammatory diseases, obesity, dementia, and higher mortality.[17] They also cause anxiety, depression, cognitive distress, and increased ruminations.[18]

If you are trying to calm your nervous system and lower RUTs while consuming a lot of highly processed foods, you are working against yourself. Look at these dietary approaches as an adjunct to your care and avoid a rigid approach. It's important to enjoy your food, as this helps create a sense of safety.

Exercise

Exercise is a key part of healing. Recommendations from the National Institute of Health and the World Health Organization suggest 150 to 300 minutes of moderate exercise each week.[19] The NIH also advises including muscle-strengthening exercises at least two days a week.[20] Even if you're completely sedentary, spending just ten minutes a day being active can provide significant benefits.[21]

The benefits are well documented and include lowering markers of systemic inflammation with a dose-related effect. The more, the better. Exercise reduces the risk of cardiac disease, diabetes, and other chronic conditions.[22] It is also associated with a significant reduction in RUTs, depression, anxiety, and chronic stress.[23] Psychological interventions provide additional benefits, but exercise alone has a strong effect on reducing mental intrusions.[24] This may be thanks to improved neuroplasticity and enhanced cognitive control through the prefrontal cortex, both of which are affected by lower inflammation.

The specific type of exercise matters less than simply doing it. Throughout my thirty-two years of clinical practice, resistance training was always a vital part of my treatment advice, and I recommended that my patients include it in their routines indefinitely. Lifting weights is a proactive way to reduce pain signals. It offers a sense of control and encourages the release of anti-inflammatory cytokines called myokines.[25] Also, as you age, you begin to lose muscle mass, a condition known as sarcopenia.[26] Strength training not only helps prevent this loss but can also reverse some of it. If you are older, and if staying independent is an important goal for you, make strength training a part of your routine.

Talk Therapy

Talk therapy—and trauma therapy, specifically—can be incredibly helpful or damaging. If you spend a lot of time rehashing your past without the aim of changing your relationship with it so you can move forward in creative new ways, your brain is developing in the wrong direction. Healing occurs by being aware of the effects of your past on your present, feeling safe, and letting go. Overanalyzing your past can reinforce your trauma story. As a physician and a pain specialist, not a talk therapist, I have learned not to encourage people to dig deeply into their past to figure out what triggered them. It is impossible to excavate all past triggers as a way to avoid all future triggers. If you are triggered, you're triggered. The main question is, "What tools can I use today to calm down?"

However, there are many different therapeutic approaches to try, along with caring, highly skilled mental health professionals who can provide effective talk therapy. The important thing is to find one who is the right match for you, and who clearly understands your goal of calming the nervous system and feeling safe today.

Choose Your Inputs Wisely

Think about what is entering your nervous system at any given moment, such as the weather, the words and behaviors of people around you, your child's cries, or your boss's demands. Most of it you can't control. However, there is much that you can control, both in terms of inputs and how we process them. There are two equally important categories of inputs to consider:

1. What are you loading into your nervous system?
2. What are you holding on to from the past?

In chapter 4, we discussed not engaging in negativity in any arena, especially criticism and gossip with close family and friends. However, considering how programmable the brain is, loading in disconcerting data from any source is problematic.

Limit your time watching the news and reading it online. The news has always thrived on a baseline level of chaos. The main difference is that, thanks to information technology, we are more exposed to it than ever before. We might feel we are in the worst of times, and we are right to be upset about major societal issues—such as climate change and political divisiveness. However, endless and obsessive media consumption drains your energy and limits what you can do about it. It also reinforces your pain circuits. You remain a victim of the world's suffering.

No one is asking you to accept or be happy about the extreme suffering in the world. However, it is important to focus on whatever is within your power to make the world a better place. Mentally taking on the totality of the misery of the world and remaining upset is a common way of remaining a victim. When you diminish your life energy this way, you cannot transcend RUTs or be a source of light to those close to you.

The only answer to this problem is to stop bingeing on negative news. Stop now and completely. There are no shortcuts and no compromises. Stop engaging in negativity of all kinds. Quit mentally taking on causes that you cannot affect or get involved in doing what you can to help. Be decisive. Sitting on the fence will only create further anxiety.

Conserve Your Energy

Heron stands in the blue estuary
Solitary, white, unmoving for hours
A fish! Quick avian darting
The prey captured

—DENG MING-DAO, *365 Tao*[27]

The heron in this poem is a powerful metaphor for how conserving our energy allows us to act decisively and quickly when we are required to do so. People become understandably frustrated when they are not healing as quickly as they would like. When this happens, one question I ask them is if they have stopped complaining about their pain and medical care, criticizing and gossiping about others, giving unasked-for advice, and taking in a constant diet of news. Invariably, they have not. At that point, they must realize that they are exhausting their nervous system, which is an absolute block to healing. Claiming a space of calm stillness, like the heron, until action is required is a clear, concrete step toward healing.

What Are You Holding on To?

Addressing anger is the most difficult aspect of healing for anyone. When I first saw patients experience dramatic healing through the Dynamic Healing method, I was inspired and felt that everyone wanted to heal. I spent hours talking to every patient about what was possible, telling them that breaking free from pain was within their reach. It was a major shock to me when, one day, I realized that not everyone wants to heal. Often, people want to hold on to their anger.

The more legitimate your anger, the harder it is to let it go. You might not want to let go of your anger toward the person or situation that harmed you. You might be spending most of your free time complaining about your traumas, engaging with pain groups, or endlessly searching for a cure. All of this is understandable. You might well be a victim and have legitimate complaints, and you feel truly and miserably trapped. Taking cognitive fusion into account, when you have become your pain, the thought of not having it can be deeply threatening.

Spite Fence

My wife and I were taking a vacation on the East Coast, enjoying a beautiful spot on a bay of the Atlantic Ocean. It could not have been more idyllic. We were being shown around the area by our hosts, and as we drove toward the end of the road, we came upon an inviting-looking community of homes. As we were commenting on the beauty of our surroundings, we came upon two large lawn signs in front of a lovely house on our left with the bay on our right. In bright red letters were the words SPITE FENCE on each sign with an arrow that pointed across the street toward a beautiful beach.

We looked to the right and saw a nice-looking fence that was about a hundred feet long and about eight feet high. It was a single partition sitting in the middle of nowhere, built solely to block the neighbor's view. Clearly, there was a feud. That was all we knew. Regardless of the reasons behind constructing this barrier, from a neuroprogramming and health perspective, this situation was a disaster.

Home is a place where we should be able to relax, enjoy our surroundings, and spend quality time with family, friends, and neighbors. However, every time those neighbors arrived at their homes, their nervous systems would activate at the sight of that fence and those lawn signs. They were prolonging a fight-or-flight state and destroying their quality of life. This is essentially what we are doing when we hold on to our anger toward someone and constantly broadcast it. The chronic state of threat physiology will eventually compromise our immune system and potentially lead to illness.

I could write a book on the topic of letting go, but instead I will ask you two questions: Why would you want to keep anything in your life that you dislike, or even despise? Why would you give that person or circumstance such deep control over you? Holding a grudge—and continually expressing a grievance—is one of the least logical things we do as humans. It is one of the most common ways we give up the power to live our lives on our own terms.

This spite fence scenario is truly a form of mortal combat. These two neighbors are physiologically destroying each other. Who will let go first? Or perhaps the real issue is, who will become seriously ill first? What eventuality will force them to focus on more important matters, such as staying alive? This spite standoff illustrates how traditional approaches to anger—reasoning, willpower, or moral arguments—fail completely.

Forgiveness

Many actions and scenarios are unforgivable, but that doesn't mean they have to keep interfering with your life today. The word *forgive* is a stumbling block for many people. What does it mean? How many people and situations do you need to forgive, and how many times? Where is the line between forgiving and suppressing? If you can forgive enough, will you heal?

Anger is a state of intense threat physiology. When you are angry, your sapiocortex is not fully functioning; you might even be blinded to your own anger. Anger is incredibly powerful, and forgiveness doesn't easily cut through all of its defenses. For this reason, instead of focusing on forgiveness, I find it much more effective to address anger by lowering your threat physiology—starting today. Calm your nervous system. That is the core issue.

Dr. Fred Luskin's book *Forgive for Good* was recommended to me in 2013 by a patient who was doing well. As I began to prescribe it as required reading, people started to heal more consistently. It is a concise and brilliant book, and a must-read for learning how to calm your physiology. It remains a core book in my healing approach. He and I are close friends and have done workshops together. We meet for lunch once a month and chat about life. One of our ongoing discussions is about the word *forgiveness*. I feel his concepts are correct, but that the techniques he recommends are simply ways to calm threat physiology. Whether or not the word *forgiveness* works for you, the underlying question is, are you willing to learn tools to effectively address your anger? Using Dr. Luskin's terminology, telling "grievance stories" and trying to enforce "unenforceable rules" are two classic ways that we hold on to our anger.

Grievance Stories

Telling the same story in which you are the victim more than three times defines a grievance story. Each time you tell it, you are reinforcing it. Many conversations center on complaining—on presenting situations that are unfair or where you have been wronged. But when you repeatedly tell a story, it becomes normalized, a fixed history in your mind. You might not hear yourself or be aware it is a problem.

Try to notice when you are repeating the same story of victimhood and stop yourself before it has solidified into a grievance story. This will be challenging at first. You must remain aware because it is such a deeply embedded pattern. If you step back and pay attention, you'll notice that we all swap grievance stories all the time. For example, when I got delayed in writing this book, I kept telling people about the pressure I felt to turn in the manuscript on time. I was happy to explain to anyone who would listen how intense it was. Then my wife reminded me I was sharing a grievance story, and she was right. I shifted the narrative to emphasize the excellent opportunity and exciting challenge of writing this book within the given time frame. What could be more fun than to learn and write about human consciousness? The stories we share with others—and ourselves—make a difference.

Unenforceable Rules

It is fine to wish someone would behave better, but most of the time, we have little or no control over their actions or the situations that give rise to them. When this wish becomes a demand in your mind, it will fester, and you might act out or say something you'll regret. Or you will remain agitated—burning up energy, firing up RUTs, and wasting your time. Instead of remaining upset with others for not meeting your standards, why not focus on yourself and your own life?

Most of your wishes for others are based on standards that exist in your mind, and you'll get triggered when they aren't met. By "triggered," I mean an input has unconsciously activated your threat physiology, causing you to react. These standards are important to you but mean nothing to someone else. You might wish your child would clean their room, get better grades, and be an honor student. Or you might want your employer to treat you and your colleagues better, and your supervisor to be nicer. Or your partner to prioritize cooking dinner over going to the gym after work. It is fine to wish these things, but when that wish becomes a demand in your mind, you are often wasting your time. You are burning energy over situations you have little to no control over. And if you try to exert control, you'll likely damage your relationship.

One example of how petty unenforceable rules can become is conflict among couples about a certain household chore. Family dynamics are powerful triggers. Out of curiosity, I asked couples in my office what annoyed them the most about each other. Over half of the couples listed how to load the dishwasher as their primary trigger, and some would begin arguing about it in my office. This is another easy way to keep your RUTs activated.

Awareness of how grievance stories and unenforceable rules trap us in negative patterns is a good start, but what do we do in those moments when anger overwhelms rational thought?

Change the Channel

There is a simple but powerful shortcut out of anger that you can use multiple times a day, indefinitely. Dr. Luskin calls it "changing the channel"; as mentioned previously, I call it "flipping the switch." Anger is the most powerful expression of your survival instincts, and you have no chance of conquering it. People spend a lifetime attempting to eradicate it from their lives, but it is not going away. We might avoid the immediate effects of anger by suppressing it in a given moment, but suppression only reinforces our anger over time, and each time it does erupt (or more subtly manifests as passive-aggressiveness), we feel guilty about it or ashamed that it keeps happening.

Anger is also powerful and addictive and challenging to let go. It triggers bursts of dopamine and other stress-related neurochemicals, providing short-term feelings of energy, power, and relief from distress—even while reinforcing destructive patterns over time.[28] But once you decide you've had enough of being a victim, you can give up the battle and go in a different direction. With awareness comes the power to change the channel or flip the switch.

For me, this approach to letting go has evolved into the "5-3-2" strategy. It is a practical tool for dealing with adversity, including RUTs. It is making the conscious decision to give up an unwinnable battle and move on. You might find yourself needing to flip the switch many times a day. Instead of saying to yourself, "I refuse to lose," change it to, "I refuse to fight." Fighting anger is like trying to yank your fingers out of a Chinese finger trap—the harder you pull, the tighter the tube constricts your fingers. Moving toward your pain allows you to escape it. Here is my version of changing the channel.

Here is the sequence of steps, with the 5-3-2 reflecting the numbers of words in each step:

1. No action in a reaction.
2. Flip the switch.
3. Move on.

5: No action in a reaction: The first step is to recognize you are angry. It may not always be obvious, so learn the disguises of anger that are common to you. Don't take any action. Say nothing. Leave the room if necessary. Take a walk. The anger may lessen quickly or last for a while. Much of it depends on how skilled you are at lowering your threat response; everyone is different. You cannot conquer anger, but don't have to let it control your actions.

3: Flip the switch: Flipping the switch means that you let your frustration drop enough to be able to think more rationally. Then, you make the decisive choice to exit the victim role. However, when you flip this switch, flip it hard. Instead of arguing with yourself that you shouldn't be a victim, or maybe this wasn't worth getting angry about, just do it.

2: Move on: Once you have returned to a rational state of mind, you'll be able to address the upsetting situation more clearly and constructively. What is interesting is that, often, what seemed so important or intolerable moments ago now disappears. Since anger is a trigger reaction within you, when you remove yourself from the situation or the person who set it off, and you are able to calm down, the "problem" can cease to exist. Instead of spending your day reacting, resolve to fully engage in your life, starting now, and move forward on your own terms.

This simple 5-3-2 approach to sudden surges of anger gets easier with practice and is remarkably effective. The same approach applies to RUTs—when you are a victim of your own thoughts, grievances, and high standards. There are many facets to anger, and many ways to process it to minimize its impact on your life. This simple 5-3-2 strategy will get you started, and it can be used at any time of day. Don't let anger run your life. Flip the switch and move on.

Choose Not to Be a Victim

Another version of changing the channel is making a deep, definitive decision not to be a victim and then spending as little time as you can in this role.

- Write on a piece of paper, "I choose not to be a victim." Date it and place it in a location where you will see it daily.
- Understand that this is a conscious choice.
- Understand that you will repeatedly fail, but at any time you can step outside this role.

- Commit to being honest with yourself; recognize your maladaptive control strategies and disguises.
- Quit "trying": "I will try" is the ultimate victim phrase. Write "try" on a piece of paper, X it out, and hang it on your refrigerator.
- Write the word "do" on another piece of paper and hang it on your bathroom mirror. (Concept from the Hoffman Process)
- Consider flipping the switch on your entire day, and then your entire life. Refuse to let anyone or anything—your RUTs and self-critical voice included—send you into reactive mode. Reclaim your power as the creative director of your life.

Self-Directed Anger

We discussed in chapter 3 how schadenfreude reduces pain by stimulating pleasure centers in the brain and releasing dopamine. Active schadenfreude manifests as bullying or TPS. The self-critical voice increases pain in a complex manner. The sapiocortex is overstimulated and dysregulated. Other pain circuits are also stimulated. The self-directed schadenfreude response occurs when the self-prediction comes true. "I knew I was a loser." "Why did I even try?" Or you might engage in self-destructive behaviors based on the need to validate your identity as a failure or undeserving. These include procrastination, showing up late for an important appointment, and engaging in risky behaviors. Again, the "failure" elicits schadenfreude. Most of this occurs below the level of your consciousness.

There are various degrees of severity in self-attack. This phenomenon operates on a spectrum ranging from mild self-critical chatter to extreme self-attack, all serving the same purpose: playing out programmed destructive patterns, which are at the core of addiction. Then the schadenfreude is a secondary response.

Self-critical chatter represents the mild end of the spectrum. This includes low-level background noise, such as "I could have done better" or "That wasn't my best work," as well as basic self-questioning. While this might seem harmless, it establishes the neural circuits for more severe forms of self-attack.

Aggressive self-attack often stems from high standards (set by family, religion, culture, employer, society, or some other authority) but is normalized self-inflicted violence. This includes setting impossible standards with harsh consequences for falling short, relentless self-criticism that never finds anything acceptable, constant self-punishment for perceived failures, and the belief that one must be perfect or worthless. What we've been taught to call "seeking excellence" is often self-bullying disguised as virtue.

Extreme self-attack is the extreme manifestation of the self-critical voice. As mentioned above, it causes more pain through self-flagellation. Schadenfreude results if your predictions come true. The neurochemicals and receptors are dysregulated, and serotonin and dopamine levels are lower, similar to a depressed state.[29]

Perfectionism: The Ultimate Victim Role

Perfectionism is the most common and pernicious form of anger. Many cultures and societies admire it as a virtue. Perfectionism fits into the anger cascade in the following manner:

- You judge a situation or a person (possibly yourself) as less than ideal.
- You blame that situation or person for being "less than perfect."
- You become a victim of "less than perfect."
- Frustration and anger consume you.

In *Ten Days to Self-Esteem*, Dr. David Burns points out that the gap between your concept of perfect and your reality is the degree of your unhappiness.[30] Perfection does not exist in the human experience. Since perfection is unattainable, why do so many of us continue to embrace it? I will offer a couple of observations from the perspective of an extreme perfectionist.

Initially, many of us were programmed to be all that we can be. We were told that pushing ourselves to the limit is the best way to accomplish this goal. Since this strategy often achieves impressive short-term results, it seems like a reasonable path. It's not. It often evolves into punishing, limitless self-criticism. For example, in the medical profession, the burnout rate among physicians is over 50 percent in every state in the United States. The burnout rate in neurosurgeons, in one study, demonstrated that it was over 65 percent.[31] The same driving energy that's pushing you up the hill will take you down far faster on the other side—and you might very well crash and burn. Striving for perfection becomes a deeply programmed pattern of thinking and behavior.

Humans will do almost anything to create and hang on to the victim role, and perfectionism feeds into this phenomenon. Since perfection is unattainable, you can remain a victim of imperfection indefinitely. It is endless self-flagellation in the form of the self-critical voice.

To understand how self-directed anger operates physiologically, consider Ashley's experience. She was a professional well on her way to healing when she picked up *Back in Control*. She saw some gaps in her process and engaged with the course and educational coaching I offer in a group setting. She experienced further improvement in her autoimmune disorder, and I became aware of her struggles with RUTs after working with her for several years. Her story demonstrates how perfectionism created chronic threat activation, and how healing required calming her physiology. Ashley's story is a classic example of self-directed schadenfreude acting as a survival strategy rooted in childhood abuse.

Ashley's Story: From Self-Destruction to Healing

Ashley's family demanded perfection, but it was never achievable. Even subpar toilet cleaning could lead to punishment. She developed a formidable defense that would define her for decades. "I mentally hated myself so badly, so severely, so horribly that nobody else could hurt me more. It was a protective reflex so that I could sit there and listen to any criticism, and I didn't care because it wasn't as bad as what I'd already done to myself."

A chaotic foundation: Instability and violence characterized Ashley's family environment. Her father was a banker whose anger was so volatile that holiday gatherings often ended with him fighting his uncle in the street until the police arrived. The responsibility for running the house fell on her mother, who lacked basic skills. Her mother became a "cardiac cripple" when Ashley was seven. Ashley had to bear responsibilities that no child should. Her parents drafted her to be the "woman of the house." All the while, she faced constant criticism for not meeting expectations.

Building the persona: Like many trauma survivors, Ashley created a persona—a carefully constructed identity designed for protection and control. "I decided who I was going to be. I created a thing that I am this, and I'm gonna make me this, and I'm going to live up to this."

This persona helped Ashley survive her childhood, and then served her well through law school and into a successful career as a high-level attorney. She became "the rock," determined that her childhood chaos would never affect her. The same drive that helped her survive abuse propelled her toward legal excellence and professional achievement.

The peak and the fall: Ashley achieved senior partner status, secured teaching opportunities, and garnered wide recognition. She was on her way to becoming a big shot in the legal world. However, success built on trauma-driven perfectionism proved fragile. The collapse began with medical crises. Ashley had been dealing with cervical cancer since she was nineteen, a consequence of being raped at age fourteen. After cancer surgery and a brief recovery, she immediately returned to demanding trial work. A severe infection soon incapacitated her, causing her to lose her position and physically scarring her. She was denied disability benefits.

Then the breakdown really started. From 2005 to 2009, Ashley experienced "the abyss"—a complete breakdown characterized by intrusive thoughts, chronic pain, and social isolation. Doctors diagnosed her with ankylosing spondylitis, a type of inflammatory arthritis affecting her spine. Now, she was suffering severe physical pain. "I was such an abject failure," Ashley remembers thinking. "How could this have happened to me? It was so unfair." The mechanism that had protected her—hating herself more than anyone else could—had now become a prison without walls. She engaged in skin-picking, finding relief in the physical self-harm while remaining completely isolated in her house, too ashamed and frightened to venture out.

The creative spark and recovery: The turning point came through purpose and creativity. Ashley began working as a public defender and later started working with the prison population. "That was the big thing that changed my life around," she explains. "I decided I was going to open my own practice and work to help other people, and I came out of the abyss."

Recovery wasn't linear. From spending time with the prison's medical personnel, Ashley learned about the effects of trauma and stress on the body. She studied neuroplasticity, the effects of trauma on the brain, and the automatic nature of intrusive thoughts. She discovered expressive writing, meditation, and Buddhist philosophy. The concept of "no self"—understanding the ego as a construct rather than reality—proved transformative.

"When I could learn that these RUTs are the ego, it's a story and not a real thing . . . that's when it made sense," Ashley reflects. "It's something I created in the past when I decided who I was going to be. I realize that this is a program running in the background, and it's nothing—it's not me, it means nothing." Her quality of life has improved dramatically.

Today, Ashley's relationship with intrusive thoughts has changed. "They're often there, but they're not distressing. They'll come and then I'll realize what they are, and just the recognition of them lets me stop and put my awareness somewhere else."

Her story illustrates several aspects of healing. The intense self-critical voice is a defense. It works for a while, until it doesn't. Engaging with others and altruism are more sustainable ways of creating safety physiology.

Summary

Healing is a dynamic process that has no end. The only destination is the present moment. Avoiding adversity while constantly striving for the future can be an effective survival strategy when you are trapped in a world of childhood chaos, as Ashley was, but it is also a surefire way to create RUTs. If you spend most of your time feeling anxious or frustrated, you are reacting to situations from the past. You are not fully present today. A fulfilling life begins by allowing yourself to feel the realities of the present moment, and then using your tools to engage, or let go, on your terms.

The concept that emotional engagement is fundamental to healing—often expressed as "you have to feel to heal"—has deep roots across therapeutic traditions. In the C-quence of healing, it is critical. However, anger and anxiety block feeling and healing through lowered metabolic activity in the higher thinking centers. It is critical to use strategies to get to the root cause that is creating symptoms instead of only treating symptoms.

The first step is learning to feel safe by addressing the output portal of the Dynamic Healing framework. You do this by directly lowering threat physiology. Methods of stimulating the PNS, primarily the vagus nerve (such as calming breathing and auditory exercises), will accomplish this.

You can also lower threat physiology through the other two portals of Dynamic Healing: inputs and processing. Diet, sleep, exercise, and calming mental health interventions all help to reduce the sensitivity of your nervous system. When it comes to the inputs into your nervous system, there are two questions to ask yourself: "What am I loading into it? And what am I holding on to?"

Endlessly fighting adversity can't work. Even if you solve some problems, countless others will follow. This will happen even without the ongoing onslaught of RUTs. Allow yourself to feel your uncomfortable emotions insofar as you can learn from them, let go, and move on. Calming your physiology will shift you from a state of threat to safety, freeing up energy to live life on your own terms.

CHAPTER 9

Soften Your Ego

According to Darwin's Origin of Species, it is not the most intellectual of the species that survives; it is not the strongest that survives; but the species that survives is the one that is able best to adapt and adjust to the changing environment in which it finds itself.

—LEON C. MEGGINSON

Remember the first time you fell in love? Maybe you had a crush on a classmate in sixth grade. What about your first true love and being head over heels to the point you felt you couldn't live without them? Your mind was full of racing thoughts and intense emotions. Your heart sank if they didn't return your phone call. This was the perfect person, and you felt whole in their presence.

People have created endless songs, books, plays, and movies about falling in love. Consider popular songs like "I'm Hooked on a Feeling," "I'm Addicted to Love," and "You've Got a Hold on Me." But this all-consuming feeling of romantic love usually only lasts a few months, maybe a couple of years. But why? Why isn't this feeling sustainable? Because it is a positive cognitive fusion, a transference reaction, and an illusion. It is based on your story about this person being "the one" who can do no wrong. We know intellectually that this is impossible. Why do we keep pursuing this fiction?

Metacognition

One reason is that this mental state really is temporary insanity. Your sapiocortex is not fully functioning; critical judgment is compromised and, in the amygdala, threat detection is suppressed when you're viewing your beloved. Being in love is also highly addictive, causing a massive dopamine surge.[1] This is positive cognitive fusion. As author Fran Lebowitz once observed, "Romantic love is mental illness. But it's a pleasurable one. It's a drug. It distorts reality, and that's the point of it."[2]

What you have lost is metacognition, which is the awareness and understanding of your own thought process. Falling in love fuses our beloved's identity with our thoughts about them. It is all we can see—for a while. What do we have left when this phase is over? If we're lucky, it evolves into true love, a long-term, unwavering commitment to another person's safety and well-being, grounded in genuine awareness. But all too often, it results in disillusionment and painful separation. Falling in love is like a migraine—it distorts your vision and makes you hypersensitive to everything, and the only cure is time.

But what happens when we apply this same fusion to ourselves? Just as romantic infatuation fuses us with fantasies about another person, we spend our lives fused with illusions about ourselves—and this fusion creates what we call ego.

Ego vs. Confidence and Self-Esteem

The process of ego formation involves this sequence: thoughts → cognitive fusion → ego → mental rigidity. Ego is a mental construct you develop to define your place in the world. Since your ego is based on approval from others (and from yourself), there is no stable point; you are never good enough, and there is no end to the pursuit. The ego is fragile and requires endless maintenance and reassurance.

Ego or identity (I use the terms interchangeably) is a manifestation of mental rigidity. Everyone possesses an ego, with varying degrees of rigidity. We create a fixed view of ourselves and defend it when challenged. We pursue an alternate reality from the vantage of our ego. Our lack of anchoring in reality compromises our ability to navigate it. Ego is a false identity based on external validation rather than authentic self-worth. I hope by the end of this chapter you'll see that protecting your identity is not only unnecessary but creates a lot of havoc.

Self-esteem is how you feel about yourself, regardless of what judgments are passed on you. You might call it self-love. Confidence arises from a realistic appraisal of your life skills and is the antithesis of ego, which often covers up your lack of skills. In the sequence of healing, cultivating confidence in the face of raw, unpleasant emotions is a necessary step. As you build the skills to manage adversity, confidence enables you to connect intimately with every aspect of your life. You can still have self-esteem without confidence. Confidence takes the form of self-compassion and the assurance that you are doing the best you can with the skills you have, considering your circumstances.

An excellent spine surgeon is not one who can perform any operation but one who has a realistic assessment of their skill set as well as their limits. If a procedure is too complicated or unfamiliar, they will refer it out. The confident spine surgeon is fully informed about the procedure, potential pitfalls, and backup. It is a sign of confidence to reach out for help, even if the person you are asking is a competitor. Confidence is grounded in reality. Ego is based on illusion.

Before you embark on any endeavor, it's important to begin with a realistic assessment of your ability to carry it out. Life is no different—it requires expertise to navigate it well. Without the expertise and confidence that come with focus and practice, you will be in over your head. Confidence comes from mastering skills through repetition and deep learning.

When we feel the need to defend and cling vigorously to an idea about ourselves, it becomes problematic. Ego is a cognitive distortion of self-labeling, and we reinforce it with more cognitive illusions. When we depend on it for protection from mental threats, there is nothing there to grab on to. As we continue to flail, it develops into an oversize, fiercely defended identity that is exhausting to maintain. We end up being *more* vulnerable to threat physiology, and *less* resilient and adaptable to what life throws at us. Authentic connection with others, and with the present moment, becomes difficult. In this chapter, we will take a closer look at the ego illusion as a driver of RUTs and threat physiology, and how we fall into its trap. Simply becoming aware of how the ego works will help to soften it. In chapter 12, using awareness as the core approach, I will present additional ways to break through its rigid confines. In doing this, we are making space and laying the groundwork to cultivate self-esteem.

The formation of the ego begins early in life, often on the playground, where the stresses that young children experience are a hotbed for anxiety, anger, and RUTs.

Power Struggles on the Playground

Living a full, enjoyable, and productive life depends on feeling safe, but when did we ever learn how? Many people grow up in chaotic households, which have been well documented to have a significant negative impact on one's life trajectory. However, schools are where defensive coping patterns become deeply rooted in young brains and provide fertile ground for RUTs.

The classroom is where students learn skills to compete in the workforce. It is competitive and always will be. The playground is where we learn social skills to navigate society. But how effective are classrooms and playgrounds for teaching us how to navigate life? Do you remember what it was like to go to school for the first time, or to switch to a new school?

First, you are leaving familiar surroundings and being thrown into a group of strangers who are just as anxious as you are. While many teachers are nurturing in the classroom, many are not. Long hours, excessive workloads, and marginal pay cause them stress. The focus is often on behavior and discipline, and the more you act out, the harsher the penalties. So instead of helping you feel safe, which would optimize the development of your sapiocortex, control tactics trap you in a cycle of fear.

Second, on the playground, you must seek approval from others to establish your identity and define your role in the world. Others have the power to withhold approval or exclude you. Using it strengthens their identity. Whether you are the one being rejected and excluded from a clique or are one of the kids in a clique that is rejecting others, you are desperately building up an ego so you can operate in this social hierarchy. What children don't realize, however, is that they are not establishing their own identity; it is being determined for them by the approval or disapproval of others. This ego is fragile and demands ongoing validation.

Third, all those competitive and judgmental thoughts that you learned in class and on the playground translate into a self-critical voice, and it is game on for RUTs. Social media and marketing add fuel to the fire: You are not measuring up, and you are missing out on what everyone else has. All too aware of your "flaws," you double down on finding areas where you can excel to create a better story about who you are. You might even rise to great heights to outrun the negativity. But you can't outrun your thoughts.

The genuine tragedy happens because of cognitive fusion, where our identity merges with our thoughts. By the time we hit middle school, we are all wearing a mask called ego. None of us knows who anyone else really is as we merge into our stories. What labels have you collected, and what armor have you put on to compensate for the negative labels?

The playground is disastrous for learning life skills. We are on the defensive from the beginning. There is little structure, with the only currency being more power and control, which manifests in multiple primitive, and sometimes, brutal ways. After all, everyone is acting out their survival instincts. Somehow, adults feel that this experience is a rite of passage where you learn to toughen up and make your own way in life. The object is to learn how to gain more power and fit in with your peers. But do you know what compassion, human connection, vulnerability, and thriving mean? Do you know how to nurture joy?

"They are just being kids." "Toughen up." "Stop being so sensitive." There is a common assumption that stress at this age is necessary and helpful. Wrong! Kids get broken and often don't recover. Then, these patterns of thought and behavior manifest throughout their lifetime and become more deeply embedded. A recent study of 682 children and adolescents found that there is no benefit gained from adversity. In fact, it leads to poor psychological functioning, lack of mental effort, and decreases in agreeableness, conscientiousness, and emotional stability in adulthood. There is no benefit to sustained stress without the capacity to process it. The authors of the study surmise that the cultural narrative has persisted because of the high-profile survivors who have excelled and broadcasted their stories.[3]

Schools must prioritize the playground as a space where students can learn essential life skills. Instead, we are taking away free time, decreasing exposure to the arts, and adding more curriculum, which further stresses students. The sapiocortex, which is the essence of deep learning, progressively shuts down, and this compromises learning. Instead of disciplining kids who are acting out, we need to determine the underlying cause and teach self-calming tools. We can teach younger generations the life skills that we, as adults, are only discovering now. Childhood patterns don't improve with time. They become more disguised and embedded.

Your sapiocortex, the region of your brain that houses your highest executive functions, starts to develop between the ages of three and seven, and continues to develop into your twenties. If you are under constant stress and seeking others' approval during these early years, this area won't develop optimally. Fortunately, the neuroplasticity of your brain enables you to create new neural circuits throughout your lifetime, provided you remain open to new ideas.

Why We Cling to Ideals

We have established that our survival thoughts and emotions are, by design, unpleasant and often disturbing. They are universal danger signals. Since they are powerful, they might make you feel ashamed, undesirable, helpless, and worthless—mainly because you have no control over them. The ongoing interaction between your body's chemistry and these thoughts ingrains them into your permanent memory, and cognitive fusion makes them feel like you. You feel compelled to create narratives about yourself to compensate for these dark sensations.

Since your unconscious brain is so powerful and never slows down, any attempt to counteract it with your ego is a losing battle. However, this doesn't stop us from continuing to try if it seems like the only option. Well-intentioned individuals often work harder to compensate for feelings of shame and worthlessness compared with those who are less reactive to these survival sensations and don't care as much.

One strategy is to identify with high ideals and take on noble causes. There is some benefit to you and others, but if you are doing it to outrun RUTs, it is not sustainable. For example, the burnout rate among activists is over 50 percent.[4] Many activists express poor mental and physical health and fatigue, and most quit the field. You are still in a chronic threat state, which means you're burning unnecessary energy. In contrast, working from a calm center allows you to sustain admirable efforts and supports healing. Giving back and altruism lower threat physiology.

Coming from a dark home environment, I defined myself by adopting high ideals and immersing myself mentally in various causes. I believed that most people lived their lives this way, and it seemed right. However, I was also judgmental of those who did not seem to share a similar approach. I will never forget the moment I read a quote from Joseph Campbell, a professor of mythology at Sarah Lawrence University: "Idealism is dangerous."[5] I was dumbfounded and couldn't grasp what he meant. Most of my thoughts and actions were rooted in ideals, and I frequently felt bad and guilty for not meeting my own internal standards. Therefore, my mind never stopped monitoring my thoughts and actions. I felt that if you didn't have ideals, you lacked substance.

I did not understand what Campbell meant until I became terribly ill. I was brought down by disruptive thoughts that arose from monitoring my adherence to my ideals. They became disturbing, intrusive, revolting, embarrassing, and invasive. There was no way I could reach my lofty goals, yet I spent most of my days countering negative thoughts with positive ones and engaging in "noble" activities to feel better. It worked for a while, but then it didn't.

Programmed for Competitiveness and Self-Criticism

While pursuing safety, peace, and companionship is fundamental to our nature, we are continuously shaped by everything and everyone around us. Unfortunately, much of this shaping affects us negatively. Those in authority commonly wield guilt, intimidation, and shame to promote better performance. We find ourselves judged and criticized. Because many of us grew up this way, it feels normal.

Parents often nag, scold, advise, and criticize their children. We're rewarded for good behavior (as defined by others) and punished for bad. Children often learn "be all you can be," which establishes unrealistic expectations and strengthens the feeling of inadequacy. We must create our own story about who we are and our place in the world to feel better about ourselves. Unfortunately, when our story is a reaction, it is not ours.

Like any living creatures, humans must compete for resources to survive. With our complex language and abstract thinking, we compete for money, achievements, power, status, appearance, knowledge, strength, and reputation. We spend much of our energy cultivating an image of strength and resilience. Instead of allowing ourselves to be vulnerable, a trait that is central to meaningful relationships, we often present a "bulletproof" persona to the world and deepen our social isolation. When we don't measure up to our competitive standards, we punish ourselves.

As mentioned in chapter 8, the self-critical voice emanates from the higher parts of the brain, but it is dysfunctional. The metabolic activity of the sapiocortex remains high, but empathy, abstract thinking, and executive function are compromised. This bullying voice in your head is a major source of RUTs. It is a cognitive strategy that you are using to counter a lifetime of negative programming. It requires so much metabolic energy that it quickly causes fatigue. Since the conscious brain is far less powerful than the unconscious brain, it is a losing battle, and it's why many incredibly competent people experience impostor syndrome. Years of early exposure to criticism will program you to hear criticism for the rest of your life (e.g., "See, you're a failure! You don't belong here!"). You will feel inadequate no matter how much reassurance you seek. This unrelenting voice will make you feel like an imposter. How long can you keep beating up on yourself while continuing to build up impenetrable walls?

Mental Rigidity

You might describe your worldview as "just the way I am," and be unaware of the effects of your rigidity. Being overly attached to your perspectives and self-image can be an early sign of developing rigidity. It's challenging to identify the moment when the ego has become so entrenched in defensive patterns that it turns problematic. Still, striving for mental flexibility is always helpful.

In one behavioral study, *rigidity* is defined as "The tendency to develop and perseverate in specific cognitive, emotional, or behavioral patterns, which are continuously employed in situations where such patterns are no longer effective."[6] Remember, mental rigidity develops for a reason; it serves a protective function. RUTs are unpleasant, often very unpleasant. By keeping your thought patterns within a narrow range of what is considered acceptable, your exposure to them lessens. This approach works—until it doesn't. This represents a form of thought suppression, and eventually, the pressure cooker blows its lid. The thoughts might become intrusive and even bizarre. Or even worse, your compensatory behaviors might become dysfunctional, aggressive, and harmful. Rigidity is a core trait of many mental health issues.

Rigidity can keep you focused and offer a framework for accomplishments, which can look like success for a time, but it is not sustainable for your health or your relationships. In the long run, you will be more productive by creating a flexible working relationship with your stress physiology.

Maintaining Your Ego

The construct of ego is a massive cognitive distortion of labeling. Every aspect of it consists of labels. Even if you have been successful in creating a solid ego, what do you do next? Ongoing effort is required to sustain it in the face of persistent negative messaging. As your thoughts become increasingly hostile through repetition, more energy is spent counteracting them. The need to build, defend, and reinforce your ego leads to racing, often disruptive thoughts, and more rigidity. Examples of self-critical thoughts include:

- I'm worthless.
- No one likes me.
- I'm not good enough.
- I'm a failure.
- Everyone else has what I want and should have.
- I'm too short/tall/fat/skinny/ugly/unattractive/unappealing.

Ironically, we use RUTs to defend ourselves against RUTs. For example, in the medical world, the pressure is intense, and physicians often have much of their identity tied up with being MDs, especially surgeons. If a patient sees a surgeon and then goes to another surgeon for surgery, the first surgeon is often upset. This might trigger racing thoughts such as *I'm not good enough*, *Why didn't they like me?*, *I'm really more competent than my competitor*, and so on. All of these are cognitive distortions defending a self-image of being a good surgeon.

Of course, the doctor has no idea why the patient decided to go elsewhere. Considerations might have included insurance coverage, proximity to care, the patient's comfort level, the choice of procedures, or possibly the nature of their interactions with the front office staff. The point is, there is no way of knowing for sure why they chose someone else, but it happened, and there is no point in spinning your wheels on a situation that is over and done with. It's okay if not everyone cares for you or your opinion. Let them find someone they feel more comfortable with. You will be better off with someone who appreciates your communication style. Once you realize you're wasting mental energy on RUTs in an effort to shore up your ego, it's easier to move on.

As we try to quiet our RUTs with more RUTs, they become ingrained and grow stronger, and the rigidity increases. The more we attach to ego, the more detached from humanity we become. We become blocked from the full range of emotions and fail to see various sides of a situation. Mental rigidity often manifests as extreme political views, irrational belief systems, harsh opinions, and deep convictions of being "right." Anything that contradicts these belief systems feels like a personal attack, causing anxiety and defensiveness. Rigidly maintaining the ego is devastating for all kinds of relationships, ranging from personal to professional. Rigidity is the antithesis of vulnerability, which is essential for meaningful interactions. Arriving at a common understanding is close to impossible. Let's take a look at the most common types of cognitive distortions we use to defend ourselves.

Cognitive Distortions

A cognitive distortion is an internal misperception of yourself or your relationship to the world that creates mental distress. These arise when your sapiocortex is not functioning optimally. They are illogical, repetitive loops formed by RUTs firing up physiology, which in turn creates more RUTs. In his book *Feeling Good*, Dr. David Burns calls them automatic negative thoughts (ANTs).[7] According to Dr. Burns, common types of ANTs include:

Labeling: putting general labels on others or yourself instead of looking at details or using descriptions.

"Should" thinking: letting "should" and "shouldn't" judgments be a beacon for your thoughts, which quickly develops into perfectionism.

Minimizing the positive: discounting your efforts or successes.

Emphasizing the negative, or "not good enough": focusing on what you don't have rather than cultivating gratitude.

Mind reading: assuming a person is thinking a certain way based on your interpretation of what they are saying or doing.

Catastrophizing: blowing things out of proportion.

Fortune telling: predicting future events based on past experiences with minimal evidence.

Emotional reasoning: assuming if it feels bad, it must be bad.

All-or-nothing thinking: failing to see the shades of gray.

Overgeneralization: assuming that a single event will keep recurring or has a broader impact than it does.

Personalization and blame: mentally taking responsibility for something you had nothing to do with.

While the ego is a cognitive distortion of labeling, whenever it feels threatened, we defend it with a flurry of additional cognitive distortions. We use the same flawed tools that created the initial problem (cognitive distortions and labels) to try to solve it. For example, let's say you identify yourself as a punctual person. Since you hold yourself to this standard, when a friend is fifteen minutes late for a lunch date, you begin to boil inside. "People should always be on time. He isn't respecting me or my time. Where is he? I'm never going out to lunch with him again." The initial distortion was that people should never be late (should thinking) or that he is disrespecting you (mind reading). Meanwhile, he was merely held up in traffic due to an accident on the freeway. Think of all the mental energy you wasted while reinforcing your RUTs.

Mind Reading

Imagine a colleague at work walks by without acknowledging your presence. You assume they are upset with you about a situation from the previous day. It's possible they just received bad news and aren't engaging with anyone.

Or recall a time when someone didn't acknowledge your email or return your phone call. You might have assumed you had upset them, or that they were unhappy with you for some other reason, when in fact they were busy or distracted. Many of us tend to mind read and project our own fears onto other people's silences.

Regardless of the context, making assumptions about what others are thinking drains emotional energy.

Should Thinking

Telling yourself how you "should" or "should not" feel and behave, whether related to current circumstances or those in the past, disconnects you from your present reality. It causes constant anxiety and disappointment with yourself and with others around you. "I should've gotten an A." "I should lose ten pounds." "I shouldn't have said that at the meeting." Then consider the number of times a day you impose these types of thoughts on other people, essentially projecting your self-judgment onto them.

Should thinking is a source of endless, needless regret about missed opportunities, costly mistakes, poor decisions, relationships, careers, and everyday missteps. It is pervasive and invasive. We are so immersed in this form of cognitive distortion that we don't recognize it as a problem.

Minimizing the Positive and Focusing on the Negative

Focusing on a partner's negative traits is harmful. The other person usually has many positive qualities that often go unnoticed. My spouse may be loving, energetic, creative, and caring. But why are they always late, or why am I the one doing the dishes? I don't like their driving. They are not meeting my needs. Over time, the story we tell ourselves about our partner can become so powerful that it can ruin an otherwise great relationship.

In my practice, I was often amazed that a patient could be 80 percent better either with or without surgery yet still be upset about their remaining problems. Even when we have an abundance of resources, we tend to focus on what we don't have. Celebrating our wins and practicing gratitude goes a long way toward calming down our nervous systems.

The Three-Column Approach

If much of our life programming consists of distortions, analyzing them is like rearranging deck chairs on the *Titanic*. We are attempting to fix a distorted thinking system with another distorted thinking system. Good luck!

Numerous approaches and cognitive-behavioral therapy tools can help create a shift in our thinking. As mentioned briefly in the previous chapter, a powerful method is the three-column technique, presented by Dr. Burns in *Feeling Good*: Write the unwanted thought in the first column, then identify the type of cognitive distortion it is in the second column. In the third column, Dr. Burns recommends writing a more rational thought. This three-column technique is a powerful tool that I have personally used to restructure my thoughts.[8]

Another version of it has evolved over my twenty years of using this strategy. By simply understanding that your unwanted thoughts are cognitive distortions, you know they are not real. In a two-column approach, simply writing your thoughts and categorizing them as types of cognitive distortions creates separation between your thoughts and your reactions to them. You can step into this space with awareness and move on with your day. There is nothing else to do after understanding that your RUTs are distortions, not real. When you don't create space for awareness, these distortions don't just maintain your ego—they become the very substance of it, creating a house of cards that's exhausting and pointless to defend.

Labeling

Labeling is a universal human activity. We are constantly labeling others and ourselves, yet no one likes to be labeled. Labeling triggers reactions and blocks awareness, detaching us from reality. Labels trigger us, and our reactions cause more intense labeling, and the chaos continues.

Epictetus was a Greek Stoic philosopher who was born into slavery circa 50 CE. In *The Art of Living,* Sharon Lebell offers an enlightening English translation of his classic work. Epictetus's insights into life were profound. One of his essays describes the difference between labels and descriptions: "It is one thing to call a person a drunk, rather than describing them as a person who drinks a lot."[9] You might not know this person or what is driving his behavior. Or if you do know him, labeling him "a drunk" blocks compassion and any awareness of the person underneath the behavior.

In modern medicine, patients often feel labeled by their doctors. Labels include "lazy," "malingerer," "drug seeker," "mentally ill," "faker," "pain patient," and many others. One seemingly benign label is a "nonsurgical problem." It requires more time to sort out a nonsurgical issue, and surgeons often shorten the visit to find patients who need surgery. Because the medical system drives physicians to be "productive" and restricts the time they can spend with you, it is not entirely their fault. To be viewed as a human being who is suffering from chronic pain is very different from being labeled a "pain patient" for whom treatments are often generalized.

The need to protect your ego can disrupt all manner of relationships—with family, friends, colleagues, and even yourself. When you are convinced that your own perspective is the most accurate and correct, it is frustrating when others disagree. It is difficult, if not impossible, to see a situation from someone else's viewpoint. You might not recognize your own inflexibility.

Negative labeling represents a particularly troubling cognitive distortion. We often use negative labels to place others in a lower category than ourselves. Much of this happens at an unconscious level. It leads us to overlook the nuances of a person or a situation. As a label repeats in our mind, it becomes as real to us as any physical object through cognitive fusion. In *The Way to Love,* Anthony de Mello emphasizes that any label, even a positive one, undermines the ability to connect with others.[10] Positive labeling can also cause us to feel less than the other person. This creates envy, which is the deepest driving force behind destructive actions.

Since your ego relies on comparing yourself with others, with whom are you comparing yourself? How many comparisons do you need to convince yourself that you are okay? When your self-image depends on others, you are at their mercy. Keep in mind that it also shores up their ego to judge you as inferior. We are constantly judging ourselves and others in an exhausting, never-ending cycle.

A related issue is gossip, which might seem harmless but can quickly escalate into something malicious. Gossip feels normal because it is so widespread and easy to engage in. However, many religions consider it akin to theft. When you gossip about someone with me, you are depriving me of the opportunity to meet and interact with that person with an open and inquiring mind. Instead, when I meet them, my unconscious mind is working to discount or reinforce the impressions I've already formed. This person has had something taken from them.

Judaism forbids gossip and views it as a major sin. *Lashon hara* is Hebrew for "evil speech" about another person, which is prohibited even if the information is correct.[11] Other religions have similar teachings. However, in today's world of social media and extremely divisive politics, slander has become commonplace. The damage inflicted and the chaos caused by malicious gossip are immeasurable, not only for the target but also for the instigators and for society at large.

Summary

There are two aspects of softening your ego while simultaneously learning to feel safe. They are separate but intertwined sets of skills. One approach is to break through your rigidity, and the other is to soften it

Always Ignore Your Enemies

I attended a five-day workshop led by Dr. Burns, whose landmark work in cognitive-behavioral therapy played a crucial role in my journey out of RUTs. I was the only orthopedic surgeon among 119 mental health professionals in attendance. Throughout the week, he emphasized the significance of letting go of your ego to connect to your true self. I came to understand my ego and idealism as a façade.

About a year later, I experienced a particularly intense set of attacks from my health care system. The hospital administration told me that I was not productive enough (based on performing procedures) and that it was not normal for a surgeon to talk to his patients. One administrator, who was my immediate boss, wanted me to stop spending so much time with my patients, despite the fact that so many of them were improving under my care. I sat in my office later that afternoon, lost in thought for over an hour. The ego-driven version of me would have quit. But Dr. Burns's words were still in my head: I realized that my colleagues were attacking their mental construct of David Hanscom, and they did not really know who I was. A burden was lifted from my shoulders, and I no longer felt the need to respond. A quote famously attributed to Oscar Wilde entered my mind: "Always ignore your enemies; nothing annoys them so much." Its origin is unclear, but I took it to heart. Why let people who don't like you make you miserable? Somehow, this phrase broke me loose.

I could not have predicted what would happen over the rest of my career. As I no longer felt the slightest need to engage with the persistent skepticism, the attacks became almost a weekly occurrence and grew more intense. I even developed compassion for my detractors, as they were the ones who were angry and upset. I was enjoying my new life. They had lost control and were escalating their efforts to pull me back into the fray.

with compassion-based methods. Both of these are centered on awareness and need to happen simultaneously. These will be discussed in detail in chapter 12.

Our basic drive is to feel safe, but the world doesn't offer much safety. For most of us, our socialization primarily occurs at school, where kids typically feel unsafe in close quarters with strangers, lacking the skills to self-regulate and get along. Ego is a mental defense against mental pain. "Sticks and stones might break my bones, but words will never hurt me" is profoundly untrue. Words literally hurt us, physiologically, and defending against them creates a lifetime of defensive thought and behavior patterns. Since everyone is looking for validation from others, our socialization process is a chaotic power struggle, dominated by the more aggressive personalities. The reactive responses become set patterns for life.

By the time you are an adult, you already have deep reactive patterns embedded in your brain, and a set ego—one that was formed to protect you from outside threats, but that you now feel compelled to defend. RUTs will continue to emanate from this destructive cycle. So, if your ego has developed from a lifetime of defensive programming, what can you do? Part of the answer is creating a more flexible ego. But you have to break through the rigidity carefully.

You can't know what you don't know—especially if you are inflexible in your thinking. You might be so attached to your identity and outlook on life that it becomes difficult to see or hear the perspectives of others. Furthermore, the more cognitively fused you are with your anxiety and RUTs, the more overwhelming it can be to try to break through them. Why would you want to break down what feels familiar and paradoxically safe? Many people don't, while at the same time feeling miserably trapped by their thoughts.

Awareness, which de Mello tells us is love itself, is the capacity that cognitive fusion destroys. It is the key to softening your ego, rebuilding your brain, and creating your new life. Ego is merely a mental construct that we can all transcend.

CHAPTER 10

Rebuild Your Brain

The only person you are destined to become is the person you decide to be.

—Widely attributed to Ralph Waldo Emerson

In the metaphor of a tree representing the C-quence of healing, connection and confidence represent the skills needed to regulate your threat physiology, but active healing occurs with creativity. The concept of healing through creativity is vital to comprehend and put into action. We are evolutionarily programmed to react and fix, not let go and embrace different experiences. But we must let go in order to move forward and create new neural circuits.

Quit Stirring the Same Pot

There is only so much of you to analyze, and only so much energy to spend on the emotions of your past before you deplete all reserves. Continuous navel-gazing can become a downward spiral. It's important to look up and take in the view. Self-focus becomes a form of mentally spinning your wheels. Research shows that there are clear limits to the benefits of inner work.[1] You cannot think your way out of a thinking problem. It has become clear to me that the only way to heal is to open up and reach upward and outward. Through new branches of creativity, new data can come in and overlay the prior data, whereas trying to fix the old data only reinforces it.

Your sapiocortex develops quickly between the ages of three and seven.[2] Think of how much children learn at this age. Almost everything is new, and children assimilate new information and experiences quickly. Why is this? Except in extreme circumstances of abuse, children have not yet built an identity or ego defense mechanism. They haven't started consciously comparing themselves with others and are wide open for learning. At some point, an identity forms in response to stress and societal cues. As they spend more time defending themselves, there is less space for learning. In chapter 9, we discussed softening your ego. Rebuilding your brain is not about creating an alternate ego. It is about opening up to possibilities and absorbing new information at face value, without bringing your ego into it at all.

Oversight of cognitive input typically occurs in the sapiocortex and represents the highest level of executive function and abstract thinking. As discussed in chapter 3, when you are in a state of threat physiology, beliefs and concepts form in the insula without rational supervision of the sapiocortex. They are "baked in" and resist contradictory facts and data.[3] These beliefs become integrated into survival identity; challenging them creates a strong threat response. Hence, a lot of RUTs. Your defensiveness increases threat physiology and beliefs become more entrenched. Rather than attempting to break into a well-defended fortress, you can use your energy to start building a new village.

Rebuilding Your Brain

In chapter 2, I introduced Dr. Robert Naviaux, a brilliant researcher who has made significant contributions regarding the role of mitochondrial dysfunction as a core trait of many chronic mental and physical disease states.[4] Remember, mitochondria are tiny structures in the cell that relay genetic signals and produce energy to keep each cell alive. The human body contains between 30 and 40 trillion cells. Under stress, the mitochondria fragment and break down. Under sustained threat, they cannot repair, and inflammatory molecules are pushed into the fluid between cells.[5] We are walking furnaces.

During one of his lectures, Dr. Naviaux displayed a provocative slide of a beautiful house, followed by a picture of the same house in flames. His point was that you cannot use the burned materials to repair the house; you must use new materials to rebuild it correctly. In other words, repairing your brain differs from rebuilding it. What you are doing by stimulating neuroplastic changes is literally rebuilding your brain. This is why anyone can heal, no matter how severe the damage. You can begin the rebuilding process right now. At some tipping point, you also change the way you process new information, and it gains momentum from there. This is how deep healing occurs.

There are many self-help books and strategies that address rumination and how to stop it. Noticing whether the thoughts are rational or not is one suggestion, but categorizing your thoughts in this way inadvertently reinforces them with focus and judgment. Snapping a rubber band on your wrist when an unwanted thought pops up is another form of categorization and negative feedback. Positive affirmations are even more problematic. In attempting to counteract the RUTs with a contradictory positive thought, you are spending even more mental energy on them. Deep psychotherapy, where you immerse yourself in your past, can also take you in the wrong direction. Lying on the therapy couch for years can deflect genuine, constructive connection with your pain. None of these approaches addresses the root cause of unrelenting threat physiology.

Cultivating the first two Cs of connection and confidence, by using many of the tools we've discussed, will allow you to spend more time in safety physiology. It's from here that you can access creativity and build a more sustainable life. Creativity occurs with action, not just learning. You must implement what you have learned and practice daily. Here are some strategies:

- Think of your life as an adventure.
- Practice altruism.
- Play.
- Get organized.
- Connect with others.

Is Life a Gift or an Adventure?

The expectation is that once a gift is given, it's yours. Attempts to take it back are met with resistance, disappointment, a sense of betrayal, and loss of trust. Once you receive a gift, you feel entitled to keep it. Life doesn't fit this criterion. It can be taken back at any time, without warning. Life is full of challenges and adversity, and it is tricky to learn who and what you can trust. It often feels like you are being betrayed. Who was it that gave you this gift? Every creature must fight to stay alive, but what kind of life is merely staying alive?

The problem isn't that life is full of challenges; it's the expectation that we should not have to deal with adversity, and then becoming angry when we experience it. This is especially true of RUTs. Where did these unwanted thoughts come from? Spending our days fighting them is not what anyone would call "the gift of life." Consider a paradigm shift where you view life as an adventure.

If you view your life as a gift you deserve, a sense of entitlement makes things worse. You are defending not only your ego but your right to live at a certain level of comfort. I recently read an article about ultrarich people who pride themselves on their discerning taste (pickiness), vociferously complain, and post their complaints online. No one is happy in this scenario—neither the complainers nor the readers of the posts.[6]

Life is an opportunity and an experience. What can you do to optimize it? Viewing it as an adventure changes the paradigm to embracing experiences that typically involve uncertainty, risk, or exploration into the unknown. The word derives from the Latin *adventurus*, meaning "about to happen" or "approaching."

Adventures take you beyond your familiar physical, intellectual, or emotional experiences. Unlike passive experiences, adventures require active participation and decision-making. Navigating adversity typically presents opportunities for personal growth, learning, and the expansion of capabilities and understanding. As you interact with new experiences, you are engaging in another form of deep learning.

The moment we understand that life is not a gift but an adventure, everything changes. This realization transforms us from passive recipients into active navigators of challenging but fascinating terrain. Likewise, the shift from a victim to an adventurer mindset revolutionizes how we approach existence. Where victims expect ease and feel resentment when difficulties arise, adventurers expect obstacles and find excitement in challenges. The victim asks, "Why me?" while the adventurer asks, "What's possible?" This reframe eliminates self-pity as a default response, replacing it with curiosity and a growth-seeking mindset.

Creativity emerges as a potent tool and an essential resource for the adventurer. Rather than trying to escape adversity—like trying to outrun a storm—skilled adventurers engage creatively with challenges, transforming obstacles into opportunities for innovation and growth. Creative engagement crowds out negative thought patterns, generating sustainable joy through meaningful activity rather than temporary relief through avoidance.

Healing is not a linear journey; the only destination is today, this present moment. Depending on the level of your stress or the state of your nervous system, you'll have good and bad days. If you label yourself a failure every time you slip or fall, you will slide back into the abyss. A more productive way to navigate your terrain is to assess your navigation skills and see where you need work. Every "bad day" is an opportunity to practice and watch how quickly you can recover. The moments, the days, the emotions, and the thoughts will keep coming. With creativity and persistence, you'll become an expert at processing adversity and nurturing joy. Progress is how well you get back on your feet.

Altruism

According to a major 2020 study out of Peking University in Beijing, China, by Dr. Yilu Wang and others, brain research shows that when you help others, you feel good and experience less physical pain.[7] Across multiple rigorous studies involving blood donors, laboratory participants, and cancer patients, researchers have consistently found that people who help others experience measurable pain relief, often within minutes of their acts of kindness. In other words, altruism—giving to someone while expecting nothing in return—is an effective pain reliever.

Using advanced brain imaging, scientists discovered that altruistic behavior activates the ventromedial prefrontal cortex (VMPFC), a region that processes meaning and significance. This activation then dampens activity in classic pain-processing areas, including the anterior cingulate cortex and bilateral insula. The more meaningful the participants found their helping behavior, the greater their pain relief, suggesting that purpose, not mere distraction, drives the effect. Brain scans also showed that the intention to help others created a preemptive analgesic state before any painful stimulus was applied. The brain prepares to suffer less when we're focused on helping others.

It is not hard to integrate meaningful volunteer opportunities, peer support programs, and community service into treatment protocols. Even simple activities, no matter how small—like calling to check in on a friend, helping your family with chores, or mowing the lawn for a neighbor—will help you feel better. When I was in college, my best friend and I would visit an elderly couple a few times a month, and in medical school, I joined the Big Brothers program. Despite my busyness, I found these regular visits quite enjoyable, and they offered me a break from the pressures of school.

A study of patients in pain from metastatic cancer showed that something as simple as cleaning common areas for ward mates (versus for yourself) produced significantly greater pain reduction. The same physical activity, but with altruistic intention, changed brain function and subjective experience. Helping with the neurological well-being of others makes us feel better. This is a biological reality. Our brains have evolved to reward behaviors that benefit the group, creating a natural alignment between moral action and personal healing. To heal ourselves, we can turn our attention toward healing others. Oddly, altruism isn't as altruistic as it sounds, and it works!

Play

A clear remedy for pain is play. I don't mean hedonism or playing to distract oneself. A better term might be *playful*.[8] You can approach any situation with a playful attitude. It helps you feel safe and taps into your creativity. Think about what percentage of your conversations with your children, partners, and friends are about current events, medical concerns, finances, and relationship issues. Instead, try to focus on what excites you. It's amazing how much time we spend in a negative headspace. Becoming aware of this is the first step toward shifting to a positive perspective. What can you change in your daily routine to make it more enjoyable or interesting?

I'm not talking about obsessive play to distract yourself. I tried that for several decades. You can't outrun your mind. Instead, playfulness is about a mindset of curiosity. By using tools to stay calm when triggered, cultivating deep gratitude, listening carefully, and removing judgment about whether a current experience is good or bad, you create space for play. This kind of play arises organically from awareness.

Parents frequently tell me how stressed they are about their children, and parental burnout is a popular news topic.[9] Meanwhile, it is almost impossible for a child to be less stressed than their parents. We have brain cells called mirror neurons.[10] When a region of your brain is simulated, a similar region will be stimulated in the brain of the person next to you. That's why laughing causes others to laugh, and why yawning is "contagious." If you are in a bad mood, you're likely to trigger a similar emotional state in those around you. You are stimulating similar neurons in the other person. Stress is bidirectional, and parents commonly blame their children for stressing them out. If you are feeling stressed for any reason, including RUTs, you are spreading that energy.

As you learn to feel safe, positive changes will happen around you. How often do you sit down and listen to your partner or child with curiosity, compared with being critical or giving advice? How much do you complain compared to sharing joy? Simply keeping a playful mindset in the forefront of your consciousness will change this energy. For years, I have asked parents and partners to listen—only listen. Nothing more. It is remarkable how hard this is to do, including for me. If you want your family to heal, *you* need to heal. Before you offer constructive criticism, pause to consider whether it is actually constructive. Often, it only causes more stress. Criticism does not make us feel safe.

There are endless ways to bring more playfulness into your life to connect better with others. You might take a morning walk, discuss a movie you both just saw, do a project or hobby together, attend a performance or sporting event. You can even adopt a positive attitude while doing household chores. It's all about your mindset and approach.

It is hard to watch a loved one suffer, and it is good to support them in constructive ways. However, if you put your life on hold until your family heals, how long is that going to take? What your family needs is for you to heal, and sharing a sense of play is a wonderful way to accomplish this.

Playing with other people stimulates the bonding hormone, oxytocin, which is powerfully anti-inflammatory. Pursuing relaxing activities on your own can also be helpful, but if you are suffering from chronic pain, there's a high chance that you are socially isolated. Even people who appear to be surrounded by friends and family often feel alienated due to the mental traps of chronic pain. Social isolation has direct, damaging effects on your health and is associated with chronic disease. Interacting playfully with others is an essential aspect of healing.

Work vs. Play

> *"This is the real secret of life—to be completely engaged with what you are doing in the here and now. And instead of calling it work, realize it is play."*
>
> —Alan Watts, American philosopher

Many years ago, I was pondering my own journey out of pain and considering some additional approaches. It hit me that the words *work* and *play* are somewhat arbitrary. I had realized that I spent my vacations trying to recover from the rigors of work and I didn't have the energy to fully enjoy myself. It became clear that much of the problem was how I viewed work and my strong reactions to the challenges of being a spine surgeon. I decided to start removing the labels of *work* and *play* from my life.

First, I loved my work and spent most of my waking hours doing it. Why call it work? Then I decided to enjoy the whole experience. I made a point of enjoying my patients, fellows, staff, and colleagues more. With this shift in mindset, my whole team relaxed. Every week, we'd discuss how to continue to improve our clinic. If someone made a mistake, no one yelled; we would sit down and calmly discuss it. Soon, my partners got involved. We had fun to the point that we would have to tone down our laughter and bantering in clinic.

One of my mentors pointed out that challenges are part of any endeavor and present an opportunity to practice coping skills. I began to embrace my work challenges head-on, with a sense of creativity. I quit complaining. As my reactions to the daily stresses dropped, I had more energy to fully engage with the day. I could write a whole book about the numerous changes that occurred in my life with that simple paradigm shift. Why not try it?

Our Workshops

My wife, my stepdaughter, and I have held seven three- and five-day workshops at the Omega Institute in Rhinebeck, New York, and one at a retreat center in Seattle, Washington. The focus of the workshops was to present the concepts in *Back in Control* in a live format. I initially thought it was a chance to educate people quickly, as I always felt the pressure of time in my clinic. What emerged was a new paradigm of community and sharing enjoyable experiences. The didactic aspect was foundational, but not what allowed people to heal. Most participants had experienced multiple disabling mental and physical symptoms for many years and felt they had tried everything. Yet, at each workshop, more than half of the participants experienced pain relief.

My approach was to create an atmosphere of feeling safe, which included sharing enjoyable experiences in a structured environment. Playfulness emerged as the primary healer. We had a tight schedule from early in the morning until the evening. About a third of it was educational, covering the principles of healing, and this was done in a large group setting. For example, Dr. Fred Luskin, author of *Forgive for Good*, was a guest speaker, and he discussed anger and took us through visualizations. Then we broke up into small groups of four or five, meeting twice a day to discuss the concepts learned during the prior session. The small groups had lunch together and stayed together for the entire workshop.

A hard and fast rule was that no one could discuss their medical care or pain. This is where I learned how much time people in pain spend complaining and discussing their medical care. Many of the participants would sneak outside to talk about their pain.

What made the workshop unique was my wife, Babs, who is a professional tap dancer, and my stepdaughter, Jasmine, who is also a dancer and skilled in performance arts. They had us learn "Cup Song," which was popularized in the movie *Pitch Perfect*. It was interesting that, with only a couple of exceptions, none of us could do the coordinated hand motions with our cups, which made us all feel vulnerable and embarrassed. But once we realized we were all in the same sinking boat, we started to laugh and throw the cups around like goofballs. Other activities included a nature walk, where participants collected objects and plants that held personal significance. After the walk, we regrouped and shared what the objects meant to us. Juggling scarves, doing somatic exercises, watching short humorous videos, and creating vision boards rounded out the weekend. As we shared these enjoyable experiences in a safe place, most participants experienced improved moods and resolved years of pain.

One year, we had a karaoke night that was quite lively. One woman on crutches got up and started dancing—without her crutches. People walking by asked what this workshop was for. When we told them it was for people in pain, they were shocked.

The bottom line is that our workshops make everyone feel safe, sometimes for the first time. One participant said the experience was like being at an adult summer camp. After years of trying everything to find relief from their pain, many people broke through it in three to five days. This happened consistently across all the workshops. This was before I had a grasp of threat versus safety physiology and the role of the PNS. I didn't understand why so many of the workshop participants were healing at rates that far exceeded anyone's expectations.

Then I met Dr. Stephen Porges and his wife, Sue Carter, who taught me about the physiology of play and social interactions. At the workshops, we had created a profound sense of safety and play, which allowed people to coregulate with each other. When they returned home to their familiar triggers, the pain returned, but their brains had reconnected with safety and play. According to self-reports, many of the participants went on to experience long-term relief.

Playfulness is an attitude that you can cultivate. You can choose to label any experience as *work* or *play*. Regaining a sense of play and curiosity about whatever you are engaged in has a profound impact on your mood and, ultimately, your pain. Sharing enjoyable or novel experiences with others enhances play.

Success Stories

One workshop participant was a middle-aged woman who had been experiencing chronic headaches for over ten years. She had also developed persistent abdominal pain and right leg pain for a couple of years. On the second day of the workshop, she noticed some rocks on the side of the garden path at the Omega Institute. For years, people had written short sayings and tributes to people they cared about on these rocks. She picked up a rock and wrote a short poem honoring her stillborn baby whom she had never gotten to see. The doctor had implied that her inadequate uterus was the problem, which caused her to feel horribly guilty. The next morning, she woke up without a headache for the first time in ten years; her leg pain and abdominal pain had also disappeared. Everyone in the group was stunned. She had no pain the rest of the week, and she remained pain-free for the couple of years I stayed in touch with her.

Another workshop participant was an older gentleman who had visited my office a month earlier for a second surgical opinion about a spine fracture from falling off his horse. He had undergone fusion from his upper thoracic spine down to the middle of his lumbar spine. He had experienced incapacitating lower-back pain for nine years and was on high-dose narcotics. The discs below his prior fusion showed minimal degeneration. The recommendation was to extend his fusion down to the pelvis, encompassing both the front and back of his spine. It was going to be a twelve-hour operation. When he arrived at the Omega workshop, he had been using the tools I outlined in *Back in Control* for a month and was already almost pain-free. His goal was to deepen his knowledge base about chronic pain. During that workshop, the rest of his pain resolved. Eleven years later, at over eighty years old, he still has no back pain and continues to toss around bales of hay.

An older business executive had been experiencing pain in her right glute area for over seven years and had difficulty sitting. She was also experiencing at least twenty-four other pain symptoms. In light of this, I told her she did not seem like a suitable candidate for the workshop because of the severity of her symptoms and the length of time she had been suffering. Most people in her situation can't or won't meaningfully engage in learning the approaches. She attended the workshop anyway and spent most of the time lying on her side. Her pain symptoms improved far more than I had anticipated, and six weeks later, her pain resolved, and she went back to work. She remarried and is still active without pain almost twelve years later.

You might think these stories are an exception. They are not. This is the reason I quit my surgical practice. I knew that the body's healing capacities far exceeded the dictates of mainstream medicine.

Get Organized

I do not consider myself an artistic person and was not raised in an environment that cultivated creativity. My wife and stepdaughter, on the other hand, have always been involved with many forms of fine art, theater, dance, and music. In a lively discussion with my stepdaughter and one of her talented friends, they asserted that being organized and artistic were mutually exclusive. I pointed out that art is almost impossible to create without some form of structure. Examine the countries where government infrastructure is deteriorating or an ongoing military rebellion is under way. When people are anxious about personal safety, they have little time or energy for creating art. The same applies to you personally. You can organize your life in a way that cultivates safety and makes space for creative endeavors.

Additionally, if you are in pain or experiencing a lot of RUTs, you are probably on an ongoing quest to find a solution to your pain. I estimate that for many people in pain, they spend over half their waking hours discussing their pain, searching online, and going from doctor to doctor in search of an elusive diagnosis. How many hours and days of your life are you spending focused on your pain rather than actively rebuilding your brain through play and creative pursuits? Are you carving out time for them?

Getting organized comes more easily to some than others, but for all of us it is a learned skill, not an inherent trait. It might help to think of living your life like running your own business. Begin with a personal business plan: Sit down and brainstorm everything that you want for your life. Let your ideas flow without stopping to analyze or organize them. Then look at your wishes in terms of your life goals. You might find it helpful to start with a vision board, where you cut pictures from magazines and select photos of what you want in your life and arrange them on a poster board. Start with reasonable expectations and avoid dramatic life changes. Set yourself up for some early wins that you can build upon once you gain momentum.

There are many organizational systems that can help you integrate healing activities into your life. Find one that works for you. One book that has been particularly helpful to me is *Getting Things Done* by David Allen.[11]

Begin Anywhere

Start small—very small. You might feel that you can't visualize or create the life you want. Don't worry about it. Just do something, anything, to start the process. Here are some suggestions, but do whatever works for you:

- Each morning, pick up a pen and pad of paper and write one goal you want to accomplish that day—just one. It can be as simple as lying in bed for fifteen minutes longer than usual and doing nothing. There is a Scottish term for this, *hurkle-durkle*. I have observed that many people in pain, especially those with RUTs, are in a hurry. Part of it is FOMO, and also the compulsion to find a cure for the pain. Moreover, our culture prizes action and accomplishment and is always in a great hurry. Slow down. Allow your body to rest. Where are we all rushing off to?
- Make yourself a healthy breakfast or reconnect with an old friend.
- Commit to ten minutes of exercise—any kind. The key is commitment and enjoying whatever level of physical activity you choose.
- Write down a few things you might do to create more order in your life. It might resemble a typical to-do list, but it's a more thoughtful set of actions. One of the to-do items could be "Set aside thirty minutes a day for self-care," which could include exercise, walking, getting outside, or another relaxing activity that you enjoy.
- Consider how much time you devote to watching TV, and what you else you can do instead. Several large studies have shown that watching TV for more than two hours a day increases inflammation, causes cardiac disease, and increases mortality.[12]
- Envision a routine you might create to center yourself and connect with your intentions for the day.

Social Connection: Oxytocin

Meaningful social connection is critical to healing. Humans evolved through cooperation and bonding. Positive interactions release oxytocin, a hormone that has high anti-inflammatory properties. Social isolation is brutal, both mentally and physiologically—I know this from both professional and personal experience. The 2025 World Health Organization Commission finds that one in six people globally is affected by loneliness, with social isolation linked to over 871,000 excess deaths per year.[13]

Along with RUTs, my social isolation was the worst part of my years in the abyss. Even the word *abyss* is not strong enough to describe the intensity of my experience. I felt isolated both when I was alone and when I was with others. Either way, my RUTs took off. A whole category of thoughts was about my feelings of worthlessness. "Why would anyone want to hang out with me?" I couldn't shake these thoughts, no matter how hard I tried to rationalize my way out of them. Nor did I have the energy or clarity to reach out for help. These thought patterns continued to spin out of control.

In 1938, Harvard researchers launched a study to investigate the factors that contribute to a fulfilling and productive life. They chose a cohort of college students, administered a questionnaire, and followed up with them every two years. The study is ongoing and is now looking at the original cohort's children and grandchildren. The most recent data was published in 2025 and, using updated AI technology, the study has evolved into a flourishing worldwide project. A key discovery is that only one factor is a consistent predictor of a good life: the quality of individuals' relationships with friends and family.

The project's current Harvard-based researchers, Robert Waldinger and Marc Schulz, recently presented the data in the book *The Good Life*.[14] The stories are compelling and show how daily choices about relationships versus material comforts can make a significant difference in life outcomes. They prompt us to ask questions like "What am I pursuing? Is it money, power, adventure, prestige, or accomplishments?" All of the stories highlight the primary role of quality relationships in a fulfilling life. Inspired by this book, I was able to dramatically lower my FOMO and concentrate more on nurturing my relationships.

Steven W. Cole, PhD, is a professor in the Division of Hematology-Oncology at the UCLA School of Medicine. His work specializes in social genomics—the study of how social environmental factors regulate human gene expression.[15] He demonstrated two factors that markedly increased the aggressiveness of white blood cells, to the point where they attacked normal cells in addition to fighting off bacteria, viruses, and other foreign invaders. They were social isolation and a hedonistic lifestyle.

His work adds depth to Dr. Sue Carter's work (mentioned in chapter 2) regarding the remarkable effects of oxytocin on health. Prior to her pioneering efforts, oxytocin was viewed primarily as a hormone associated with pregnancy and lactation. Her efforts highlighted its role in social bonding and its anti-inflammatory properties. Dr. Carter has coined the term *sociostasis*.[16] It refers to the regulation and maintenance of physiological and psychological stability through social relationships, rather than in isolation. She describes it as the process by which individuals return to a stable baseline or equilibrium, specifically in the context of relationships—emphasizing that true physiological balance (homeostasis) cannot occur alone but is achieved through social connection and interaction.

Both Dr. Cole and Dr. Carter are pioneers in their respective fields, and their findings are remarkably complementary. They have both found that there is a bidirectional relationship between social isolation and chronic pain, with a slant toward pain being the initial event. This link aligns with the fact that a high percentage of patients in my surgical practice were socially isolated or lonely. This was often the case even when patients were living with their families. It is challenging to reach out when you are in pain, and it is easy to push people away by complaining and being in a bad mood.

One paper looked at 105 married couples with one spouse in each couple suffering from chronic pain.[17] Each of them wore a monitor. When the spouse in pain complained or exhibited pain behavior, the other one would have a predictably hostile response, including in their physiological reaction. Then the person in pain would have increased pain for over three hours. Interestingly, the person in pain kept complaining despite it causing more pain. I see this interaction as a "chronic pain marriage-go-round." Your spouse, whom you need for support, becomes a source of more pain.

I noticed on my patients' follow-up questionnaires that they frequently checked off reconnecting with family and friends as a significant component of healing. This requires being vulnerable, which is challenging when you feel trapped and angry. Actively connecting with family and friends is a critical aspect of healing. Oxytocin, according to Dr. Carter, is nature's healing medicine.

Racket Sports

One way of establishing social connections is playing a sport that requires regular social interaction. Playing racket sports is an especially effective intervention that calms and reroutes the nervous system. As part of my self-directed course, The DOC Journey, I hold one-hour virtual group Q&A sessions twice a week. One woman who is a participant in these sessions has experienced a nice decrease in RUTs over the course of a year. A significant breakthrough in her relationship with her daughter happened through playing badminton. In a recent session, I pointed out that when she first joined the group a year ago, she never smiled; now she never stops smiling.

My wife and I started to play table tennis in our backyard about five years ago. We quickly discovered how relaxing it was, even for ten to fifteen minutes. It is also social, and any level of player can grab a paddle and keep the ball in play. I have been playing since I was eight years old. My father was a hardworking physician and wasn't home much. But even when he was dead tired, he would play table tennis with his four children. It was one of our most enjoyable family activities.

About two years ago, my wife and I started playing doubles at our health club with eight other people. We play twice a week and have enjoyed getting to know the members of the group. What is nice at this stage of life is that none of us cares whether we win or lose, and we laugh a lot. I was not aware of the health benefits of racket sports until I looked them up.

The sports that have been extensively researched are table tennis, tennis, racquetball, and badminton.[18] Research has shown that playing regularly adds about seven to nine years to your life with a significant improvement in cognitive function. Tennis seems to have the most significant impact, but all of them have similar benefits. I assume pickleball is in the mix, but it is a relatively new sport for which I did not find a study.

Most of the data is from adult studies, but one regarding young children caught my attention: It is concluded that longer experience with tennis was associated with better performance in working memory and cognitive flexibility in children between the ages of eight and twelve. Furthermore, tennis experience is positively related to executive functions. The results of the present study might have significant practical implications for parents and educational settings in designing physical activity programs to improve cognitive function in children.[19]

Racket sports challenge mental quickness, improve hand-eye coordination, promote social connection, and provide full-body exercise. Years ago, the data showed these sports to be so impactful and readily accessible that the NIH felt they should be initiated as a public health effort. Unfortunately, that did not happen.

Summary

We are born as open and impressionable creatures, full of curiosity, playfulness, and an eagerness to learn. There are innumerable sources of learning, and we trust our elders to teach us about the world—how to navigate it safely, joyfully, and productively. Learning words and concepts is essential, but imitating actions is a more powerful way of learning.

But what often happens? In a protected and nurturing environment, our light might remain bright for many years, sometimes indefinitely. But for many of us, the light becomes progressively dimmer, and at some point, we tip into the abyss of chronic mental and physical pain. The light is extinguished, and it is a dark place without hope of escape.

Darkness disappears with light. You can flip the switch and turn on the lights. But first, you must find the switch, and that is where your upbringing might have let you down. The switch is inside you. If you have never felt safe and have normalized your suffering, why would you look for it there? Perhaps you are so locked inside your suffering, so busy fighting darkness, that you are too tired to try. Or maybe the light frightens you because it is so unfamiliar.

The good news is that it's never too late to turn on the light and rebuild your brain in any way you choose. The first two C's of the healing C-quence, connection and confidence, are your new processing system. With your deeply rooted skill set, you can break up the rigidity of your ego defenses and reconnect with the present in safety physiology. This allows for the definitive C of creativity to happen, where you consciously choose your inputs and create new neural pathways. Here are some ways to load in new data and move forward with your life:

- Reconnect with the best parts of who you are.
- Cultivate compassion for yourself and others.
- Nurture gratitude.
- Re-engage with an interest or hobby that once brought you joy.
- Take up a new interest or hobby (e.g., painting, music, dance, sports).
- Spend quality time with family and friends.
- Get out in nature.
- Spend time with a pet.
- Step outside your own perspective by listening deeply to others.
- Create a detailed vision of how you want your life to look.
- Get organized so you are able to start executing your vision.
- Connect to the larger picture of existence through religious, philosophical, or spiritual practice.

Cultivating a healthy root system will ground and energize you, while mastering calming skills will restore a sense of safety and build up your confidence. But true growth and healing occur at the top of the tree—through the light-seeking branches of creativity, not in root analysis. After spending so much time in the dark, you must look up and out to bring new data into the brain. Stop stirring the same old pot. Bring playfulness, altruism, curiosity, and gratitude into your life and treat them like learned skills. Remember, your brain will develop wherever you place attention. Where will you place it next?

Part Four

Your New Life

CHAPTER 11

Awareness Is All You Need

Love is awareness. When you are aware of what is, you love it. When you are not aware, you hate it or are indifferent to it.

—ANTHONY DE MELLO

Anthony de Mello (1931–1987) was an Indian Jesuit priest, psychotherapist, and spiritual teacher who developed a unique synthesis of Eastern and Western spiritual traditions. He was a brilliant writer who passed away before the rise of modern neuroscience. Many years ago, a colleague of mine gave me his *The Way to Love.*[1] The book pierces through many layers of the identity we try to create. He defines love as awareness. I resisted this idea for many years, but now I strongly agree with him. From a neuroscience perspective, I understand that when you are in a state of survival, you are no longer fully present in the moment. We also develop a lifetime of patterns that keep us in this state. Awareness cuts through them. His book has become one of the key references for the healing process that I have developed with my patients.

Awareness, compassion, and *love* are words that describe the same state of being. You are fully present in the moment without judgment. As your healing journey unfolds, you'll discover that there is only one word you need to heal: *awareness.* Metacognition, or thinking about thinking, is most effective in this state because your sapiocortex is functioning optimally. In this space, you are completely alive and human.

Unfortunately, the gift of complex language that enables metacognition also traps us as we develop our ego. Sadly, the ego becomes a rigid identity that we fiercely defend. This ongoing struggle reduces the function of higher thinking centers and hampers metacognition. Eventually, we become prisoners of our powerful ego, which is made up of endless RUTs. Then, through cognitive fusion, we identify with our thoughts and stories, most of which are cognitive distortions. What a tangled mess! Fortunately, a simple solution exists for this complex problem.

Awareness dissolves cognitive fusion, creating space for you to reset your nervous system. It also helps you sit with your thoughts instead of reacting to them. Remember, thoughts are powerless; it's our reactions to them that give them energy. While de Mello described awareness as a single, unified state, in practice I've found it helpful to recognize different doorways into this state. Each person might find certain approaches more accessible than others, but they all lead to the same destination—being present in the moment.

Awareness in Action

Awareness is the key that allows us to go beyond our thoughts. How is this possible? Can it really be this simple? It sounds unlikely. Awareness works on many levels, and people use it in different ways. The first step in developing deeper awareness is noticing when we are operating on autopilot. Most of our daily actions and reactions happen automatically; we're basically sleepwalking through our responses to life. Awareness is the moment you wake up mid-sentence and realize you're engaging in gossip or catch yourself mid-judgment, recognizing you're labeling someone based on limited information. It's the difference between reacting without thinking and responding intentionally.

Awareness helps us grasp the details of a specific threat. Too often, we quickly label a challenge as unsolvable and give up before genuinely trying to solve it. We make major decisions without fully understanding the situation, especially regarding our health. We assign mental labels like "too difficult" or "not worth the effort." Even worse, we often label people. We project our version of their actions and words onto them, and as a result, we don't truly know who they are as individuals. What about societies and groups of people? Labeling them as "less than" dehumanizes them and justifies evil acts.

Embarking on a significant project, such as constructing a skyscraper or developing a powerful computer, requires understanding even the smallest details. This is crucial both in the design phase and when solving problems. The human body is far more complex than any man-made machine, and chronic illness involves many components that are unique to each individual. Understanding yourself, your environment, and your coping skills is fundamental and essential for healing. Similarly, the most effective doctors take the time to know a patient beyond the presenting symptoms.

Being aware is much more engaging than forcing your opinions on others, and it requires less effort. Constantly imposing your worldview on anyone willing to listen can become exhausting. You already know what you think, but why not take a moment to relax, listen, and let your world expand?

We are clear about what we don't want, and it's easy to complain. But what do you want? What do you truly want? When will you decide to stop fighting RUTs and start actively living your life? Awareness is the key. As you practice the healing strategies in this book, they will become habits. Over time, awareness will grow, and your body will handle the rest.

Four Types of Awareness

Through my years of clinical practice and personal experience, I've observed that awareness manifests in distinct but interconnected ways—showing different ways we lose touch with the present moment and, more importantly, how we can reconnect. Here are four types of awareness to consider:

- sensory
- emotional
- judgmental storytelling
- ingrained pattern

Sensory Awareness

Sensory awareness involves paying close attention to the tangible, sensory details of the present moment—such as the texture of objects, subtle variations in color, the rhythm of repeated movements, and the quality of sounds. It's not just mindfulness but a specific focus on external physical details and sensory inputs rather than internal experiences.

Think about how you feel when you're deeply involved in a favorite activity. It might be knitting, gardening, performing, cooking, writing, hiking, playing a sport, learning a new skill, solving a crossword puzzle, or creating art. I'm an amateur bird-watcher, and the only time my wife says I am relaxed is when I am bird-watching. I find it calming to be out in nature, and paying attention to the intricate beauty of birds in their natural habitat draws me in.

Focusing on the details of what you are doing right now crowds out RUTs. Connecting to every sensation of any activity, including work and household chores, helps you achieve this. I vividly remember a patient I saw about five years into my surgical practice: a disabled veteran whose pain diagram showed he experienced constant uncomfortable sensations throughout his body. He was a large, muscular man in his mid-forties. His hobby was building motorcycles, specifically choppers. He showed me some pictures; they were beautiful machines. They looked as good as the ones I saw in the documentary *Motorcycle Mania*. He was talented and dedicated a lot of time and effort to his hobby.[2]

After reviewing his imaging studies, I found no anatomical reasons for his symptoms. As a young surgeon with limited knowledge of chronic pain, I had no answers. I confirmed he had completed all his tests and told him that surgery wasn't a good option. Just as I was about to get up and leave, he suddenly leaned forward and said, "You know, Doc, when I am in my shop working on my choppers, I don't feel any pain." At that moment, I did not understand how this was possible.

You might say, "This is true for physical pain, but I want to know about RUTs." Remember, they are different manifestations of the same underlying threat response. During the last five years of my fifteen years in the abyss, my RUTs were intense. However, they did not bother me during surgery, when I was focused on every move. It was when I was less present that they worsened. Recognizing this dramatic difference eventually helped me see it is possible to crowd out negative thoughts with environmental awareness.

A Mentor Who Puzzles

A few years ago, one of my mentors shared that before starting a major business project, he would work on a complex jigsaw puzzle. He believed that the sustained hand-eye coordination, along with the challenge of completing the puzzle, helped him to relax and organize his thoughts. Many ideas came to him while assembling these puzzles. He was well known in his field for developing highly innovative business opportunities that others couldn't imagine. He had an exceptional talent for finding solutions where others only saw problems.

Curious, I started my own puzzle journey, an awareness practice I found both calming and mentally engaging. One particular puzzle required me to use a technique I had used in surgery for many years, highlighting its importance in managing stress, especially regarding RUTs. It involved paying close attention to even the smallest details of the pieces—colors, shades, patterns, sizes, shapes—rather than fixating on the outcome.

The Rainbow Challenge: From Fight to Flow

One day, while I was deeply focused on writing this book, my wife brought home a jigsaw puzzle. It was a thoughtful gift she had given me with good intentions. However, as soon as I opened it, I silently groaned. It contained 1,000 pieces, featuring a circular rainbow pattern with colors blending into one another. It clearly seemed designed to frustrate anyone brave enough to try it, and I didn't have much time. It sat in the corner for a few weeks.

One evening, I decided to take a break and spend a few minutes on the puzzle. When I dumped the pieces onto the table, my brain immediately labeled the task: "This puzzle is too hard. It's not a good puzzle. I'll never get it done. Why am I wasting my time?" I felt my body tighten. Despite my resistance, I started with what seemed to be the only logical approach—finding the edge pieces. Even this proved challenging. The patterns were so similar that I could barely tell the difference between the edges for each side of the puzzle. The circular rainbow pattern meant colors wrapped around continuously, providing no clear landmarks. Each time I looked at the picture on the box, it offered little help. After struggling for an hour with minimal progress, frustration fully set in. I was about to accept my initial assessment of the puzzle: unsolvable.

Instead of quitting, I instinctively changed my approach and stopped referencing the picture. I shifted to observing overall patterns and focusing on each piece. I noticed unique shapes, subtle shade variations in color, and tiny patterns within the rainbow gradient. I assembled small clusters of two, three, sometimes four pieces. I didn't try to place them in the larger puzzle. I was creating islands of certainty in a sea of confusion. One corner gradually took shape. I continued to work from the known to the unknown, moving from the inside out. Then, something unexpected happened: I began to notice incredibly subtle details that had been invisible to me before—minute dotted lines in some pieces, dashed lines in others, nearly imperceptible variations in the hue of adjacent colors, and tiny flecks of color that distinguished one part of the spectrum from another.

Instead of sorting pieces into many categories, I let my brain absorb the entire puzzle and recognize patterns I couldn't consciously explain. Some moments felt almost magical—I'd pick up a piece meant for one section and find myself placing it in a completely different one. As my attention to detail increased, the puzzle came together faster. What once seemed painfully slow now felt smooth and natural. Pieces that initially confused me now seemed to reveal their proper places almost on their own.

After about ten hours spread over several days, I experienced something transcendent—a state of immersion that athletes and artists often call "being in the zone" or "flow." It reminded me of something I read in Daniel Levitin's book *I Heard There Was a Secret Chord*, where he explains how professional musicians who have practiced extensively reach a point where "the music plays itself, and you're just going along for the ride."[3] That's exactly what happened. I became completely immersed in the puzzle, experiencing a strong sensation of watching my hands move almost automatically, outside of my conscious control. Pieces clicked into place effortlessly. I wasn't actively thinking but rather observing and feeling. This state, where intense focus paradoxically boosts a more holistic and intuitive understanding, is the most effective problem-solving mode humans can achieve. The puzzle I initially thought was impossible was halfway finished in a few days. I had to intentionally pause to finish writing this book. The emerging picture was truly beautiful, but the real beauty was in how my approach and attitude changed throughout the process.

Being in a flow state occupies your mind enough to reduce RUTs. The big question is whether you can reach this state regardless of how good or bad your day is. Being in the flow with negativity is as important as connecting to positivity. With deliberate practice, it is achievable. While environmental awareness teaches us to focus on external details, there's another level of awareness that many find more challenging: turning that same level of attention inward to our emotional landscape.

Emotional Awareness

Emotional awareness is both the biggest challenge and the best opportunity for healing. It involves deeply understanding how and what you feel. We strongly dislike being in a threat state for a long time. We crave safety and get frustrated when we can't find it. Feelings, not thoughts, guide our behavior.

Why is there such a barrier to experiencing deep emotions? It originates from our evolution. Being vulnerable—physically or emotionally—is not advantageous in nature. It's essentially a matter of survival of the fittest, where vulnerability often results in danger. We see the fate of the weakest hen in a chicken coop. Humans are wired with the same survival instincts.

But there is a strong incentive for training yourself to feel. Awareness and emotional vulnerability are essential for successful relationships in all areas of your life. Emotional awareness is a challenging skill to develop. It requires figuring out who you can truly trust. Naturally, it requires some risk to place your trust in someone, and a betrayal of your trust can cause profound and lasting pain. So, what should you do? Learning to be vulnerable means allowing yourself to experience pain, processing it, and then moving forward. Many people give up trying, and others never begin—missing opportunities to find and sustain meaningful relationships. What about you and your self-critical voice? Can you trust yourself?

This is why being raised in an abusive family environment is so damaging. If the people whom you counted on to care for and nurture you broke your trust, how can you allow yourself to be emotionally aware and vulnerable? Like a feral cat that has only ever survived on its own, you might not even know what it feels like to be safe. Your hypervigilance will only grow as life gets more complicated.

Emotional awareness is a learned skill that can be challenging for anyone, regardless of upbringing. But with practice, anyone can cultivate awareness of their emotional landscape.

Feel to Heal: Pendulation

Mind over matter and positive thinking don't work because they block connection to your emotions. Repressing or suppressing painful emotions will not free you from their grip. You must "feel to heal." However, if you were suddenly exposed to the full force of your painful emotions, it would be unbearable. The pain would be too intense. An alternative approach, coined by Dr. Peter Levine, is a process called "pendulation," where you allow yourself to be exposed to a manageable level of emotions, then pull back and re-engage when you're physiologically ready.[4] It's a lifelong process that always honors your tolerance level to unpleasant emotions. Some days you can tolerate more than others. Be nice to yourself. Don't try to fight through a bad day. Let it happen, use the tools you can, and move on when you feel better. Over time, you'll be able to tolerate more and process emotions more easily. However, survival emotions are deeply unpleasant, and that will not change. It is again the reason you must assess your skills rather than monitor your progress.

Pursuing the path of self-discovery can be painful. We often put a lot of energy into feeling good to avoid feeling bad, but life will always present additional challenges. A more sustainable approach is to learn how to tolerate the bad and allow the good to surface.

Compassion-Focused Therapy

Given the intensity of these emotional challenges, researchers have developed specific therapeutic approaches to help people navigate their inner landscapes with less suffering. Dr. Paul Gilbert is a British clinical psychologist, researcher, and professor of clinical psychology at the University of Derby.[5] He is the founder of compassion-focused therapy (CFT), which was officially developed in the early 2000s. He created it to address self-criticism and shame loops, which are at the core of RUTs. Compassion can calm the threat response. Anger and anxiety block awareness, but awareness can break through this barrier. To understand how compassion can regulate our threat response, it helps to have a visual framework for our emotional states.

I attended a compassion conference hosted by the Charter for Compassion in Louisville, Kentucky, in 2013. I met Dr. Chris Irons, a British clinical psychologist and collaborator of Dr. Gilbert's. His lecture introduced CFT, emphasizing that three core categories of emotions are central to the human experience. He showed a slide with three colored circles arranged in a triangle. There were bidirectional arrows between each, illustrating how people shift among three emotional states. Remember, emotions are feelings that reflect your physiological state:

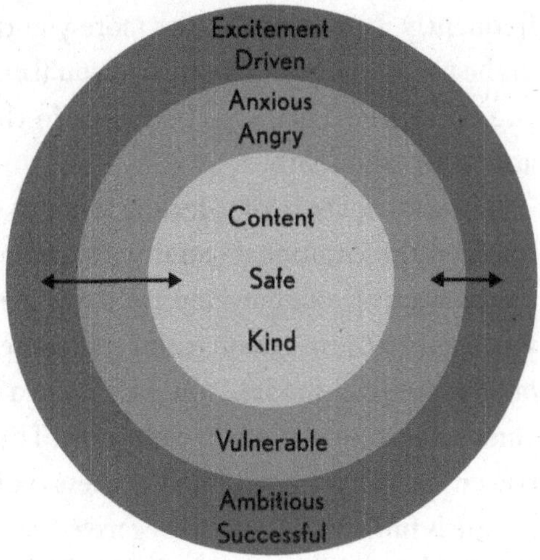

- **Red (represented by the medium-grey second inner ring):** threat and self-protection; threat physiology (fear, anxiety, anger, shame)
- **Blue (represented by the dark grey outer ring):** doing and achieving; mixture of threat and safety (pleasure, achievement, excitement)
- **Green (represented by the light grey center of the circle):** safety and recuperation; safety physiology (affection, contentment, social bonding)

The diagram made sense to me. I was excited about the conceptual model and showed it to my stepdaughter, Jasmine, who, at twenty-one, was wise beyond her years. She looked at it for a while and said, "These should be in circles." After some thought, I understood her point. Here's what it looks like: three concentric circles, green at the center, encircled by a red "ring of fire," and a blue perimeter. The message is that all three are necessary parts of life. The therapy encourages self-compassion, regardless of emotional state. Here are some reasons I agree that the concept is best illustrated as concentric circles.

Life in the Green, Red, and Blue

The green circle in the center represents the place where we believe we should spend most of our time. While it's essential to devote as much time as possible to resting and regenerating, that is not what life is about. Life is inherently challenging, and stressors keep coming at us. Using your unique set of coping and healing strategies, you'll be able to find peace of mind frequently. Paradoxically, the more you try to stay unwaveringly centered in the green, the more frustration you'll experience when something pushes you off-center. Then, you'll be back in the cycle of anxiety, self-criticism, and racing thoughts.

The goal of Dynamic Healing is not to stay in the center, but to navigate between the emotional states with awareness and on your own terms. By being aware of your emotions, you can use your skills to choose which color you want to be in—green (calm and centered), blue (active and achieving), or red (survival mode). You only have a choice if you are aware of what emotional state you are in right now. This conceptual diagram of concentric circles can be a helpful awareness tool.

Life is full of positive and negative challenges. It is exciting and dynamic. While it is important to find time for rest and recuperation in the green center, it is in the blue ring that we lead the majority of our lives. We need adrenaline, cortisol, and other chemicals to mobilize us. You might be an adrenaline junkie who feels the most productive in the red ring of fire, which can be effective in reaching goals or during high-pressure situations, but no one can stay there for long without burning out or falling ill.

Life in the blue, however, means fully engaging with whatever is right in front of you in the moment, pleasant or unpleasant. For example, you're on vacation, sunbathing, exercising, engaging in new adventures, and having a great time. You feel relaxed and aware that you're safely in the green zone. Now you need to pack, travel, unpack, and return to your daily routine. You might not notice, but it requires crossing the red ring to get into the blue zone of activity and alertness to accomplish these tasks. Any number of tasks, such as preparing to start a new project or even crossing the street, require a mixture of threat and safety. We have little choice in which ring we end up in a given moment. It is your body reacting to cues of threat and safety, with conscious thought following one to ten seconds later (as described in chapter 2). With awareness, we have a lot of more agency and access to strategies.

Another way of thinking about it is Anthony de Mello's idea that awareness breaks through the layers of protective ego we build up. It can be painful to pass through the ring of fire of threat physiology—until it isn't. As you soften your ego and train yourself to be nonreactive to your survival emotions, activities like going on a date, navigating a city, or performing in front of an audience become routine, and the red ring shrinks. This allows you to move with skillful awareness between emotional states as necessary, maximizing your time in the blue. Unfortunately, many of us spend a lot of time in the red worrying about almost anything. We needlessly burn a lot of extra energy. Life in the blue is much more fun.

THE RING OF FIRE

Unfortunately, many of us don't truly know what green (safety) feels like. Too many of us subscribe to a system of reward and punishment. When your foundational environment from early childhood is marked by anger and chaos, that green circle might be very small, or even nonexistent. How safe did you feel as a child? How often were you exposed to people arguing or fighting? How do you react when you're criticized, or when you are constantly held to impossible standards? What was it like to experience punishment, especially when you believed it was unwarranted? Even if you felt safe at home, what was school like? Were you bullied? Were you a bully? Even if you manage to establish physical safety, stressful situations and RUTs will keep coming back.

It's easy to get stuck in the red. When you've spent so much of your life battling hardship instead of feeling cared for and safe, you might not know how to get out, or that getting out is an option. In India, when elephants are small, trainers typically chain one of their feet to a stake to teach them to stay in one place. When they grow into large adults, they could break their chains or pull out the stake with minimal effort. However, since they have been conditioned from a young age not to resist the constraint, when they feel the chain pulling, they stop trying. The adult elephants still believe the small stake is unbreakable. Anger is similar because it anchors you down, preventing you from moving forward. Recognizing the nature of this bond allows you to break it. But now that you're an adult, learning how to shift from threat physiology to safety physiology is your responsibility, and yours alone.

Anxiety is a fundamental physiological state. You wouldn't be alive without it. No matter what activity you're doing, it's always present. Anxiety follows a gradual progression from alertness to nervousness, fear, anger, panic, paranoia, and terror. It's so common that you might not even realize how much anxiety is fueling your thoughts. You might say to yourself,

"I'm not anxious" or "I'm not angry." Think again. You are alive, and these emotions help keep you alive. Everyone carries anxiety and anger, and suppressing them triggers your body's stress response. It's like being stuck in quicksand: Fighting your emotions makes you sink faster into them, when the solution is to relax and float.

The ring of fire is not where we want to live. Many of us work very hard to stay in the blue and out of the red by creating a life that is enjoyable, busy, interesting, and stimulating. Sustaining a high level of activity can be both productive and destructive. Many of us keep busy in a constant effort to avoid the red, without realizing that anxiety is what's fueling us and that we're in fact falling into the red zone.

You might ask, "Why not stay in the green?" Good question. It seems like a great place to be, and some people are more able to enjoy it than others. However, it requires that you stop taking risks. When you stop trying new things and forging new relationships, your world shrinks, and you become less tolerant of any time that you have to spend in the red. Life in the green can also become a trap.

Every emotion you feel results from a complex interaction of hormones and neurotransmitters. The boundaries between them are not always clear. However, the circles of green, red, and blue serve as a helpful tool to quickly check in with yourself during the day and evaluate your emotional state. Practicing non-judgment, regardless of your emotional state, is fundamental to healing.

Implementing Compassion-Focused Therapy

CFT continues to expand and is becoming part of mainstream medical thinking. I will share some self-guided concepts to help you progress.[6] However, I recommend seeking more comprehensive and structured resources if you feel stuck. CFT methods are among the most effective for RUTs, as well as for other mental health concerns.

Cultivate self-compassion. Compassion, love, and awareness have the same root. Compassion is a form of awareness. Awareness dissolves the ego, so theoretically, there would be no need for self-compassion. However, few of us will ever reach nirvana, so let's meet ourselves in the present: We all have egos. Defending them creates RUTs. Softening the ego lowers RUTs, but it still needs care. Rather than defending the ego, we can treat it with compassion. Compassion is a direct response to the self-critical voice. Neither building up your ego nor reassuring yourself about the labels you've attached to yourself will help you out of anxiety, anger, or RUTs. Having compassion for yourself (rather than self-aggrandizement or self-pity) brings instant relief. According to Dr. Gilbert's framework, there are three pillars of self-compassion that dissolve your attachment to ego:

Self-kindness versus self-criticism: Replace the bully in your brain with a buddy.

Common humanity versus isolation: Keep in mind that we all suffer, regardless of our circumstances.

Mindful awareness versus cognitive fusion: Connect with your unique values instead of manifesting what others think you should be.

SELF-KINDNESS

A powerful way to break free from judgment is to *silently* wish people well. In the previously described sessions I hold in conjunction with my course, I frequently encourage participants to do this—with anyone, but especially with those who irritate or anger them.

You don't need to verbalize your good wishes or change your hostile feelings. You have a right to be angry, but how long do you want to give up the quality of your day to someone you dislike or are upset with? If you witness that person failing at something, you will have the pleasure of feeling that justice has been done (schadenfreude). This is all normal survival physiology in action, along with mental mechanics.

Wishing someone well is another form of flipping the switch and moving on, and it is a countermeasure for schadenfreude. Usually, your judgment of that person is based on your interpretation of what is correct behavior, but it is yours alone. Since your judgments (labels) reflect your self-judgment, you'll see what is in your mind and hear your self-critical voice. So, when you wish that person well, in a sense you are actually wishing yourself well. When I do this exercise, I like to add, "That person is doing the best they can based on their skill set and circumstances." It is a remarkably effective self-compassion exercise. People find it difficult to do at first, but it gets easier with practice.

This exercise isn't completely altruistic—it's highly beneficial for the person doing it. Your thoughts influence how your brain is wired. A compassionate outlook rewires your brain to see the world (and yourself) in a more positive light. Instead of fighting evil thoughts, you are building more enjoyable neural circuits. You can reinforce this exercise by periodically placing your hand over your heart as you cultivate compassion. When you are kind to yourself, you can more easily extend that kindness to others.

Our Common Humanity

Your self-critical voice is so ingrained that you might not even notice it. Take a moment to gently remind yourself that being human means having inherent limitations. At the very least, none of us is getting out alive. We are the only species capable of this kind of self-awareness or metacognition. Aren't you empathetic when someone is facing a severe loss, or just going through a rough time? Can you connect to similar empathy for yourself? We share a common experience: consciousness.

In *The Art of Happiness*, the Dalai Lama makes a powerful point: We often compare ourselves with those who have more than we do. Why not compare yourself with those who have less?[7] Remember, envy is a normal survival response. Of course, you want more than what you already have—this is an evolutionary instinct to increase your chances of staying alive. Suppressing envy can cause chaos in your brain, and it's a surefire way to trigger RUTs. Recognize it, detach yourself from it with awareness, and move forward. Actively appreciate what you have. Nurturing gratitude is a corollary of remembering our common humanity.

Judgmental Storytelling

Your brain acts as a storytelling machine, and most of the stories it creates are fictional. Remember those cognitive distortions we discussed earlier? They don't just cause temporary confusion and then fade away. Instead, they serve as the raw material for building your entire identity. A fleeting thought like "I'm not good enough" can turn into the main theme of your life story. A moment of disappointment might become "People can't be trusted"—a core belief system.

You build an ego by weaving distorted thoughts into seemingly coherent narratives about who you are and how the world works. The irony is that the stronger your ego, the more fragile you become. When someone challenges your carefully constructed identity, you don't only feel criticized—you feel like you're dying, because in a sense, you are. The "you" that you've spent years building is under attack.

But you don't need to fix these hardwired circuits. You simply need to recognize them. By nurturing awareness of distortions without fighting or judging them, something magical happens. You create space between yourself and your thoughts and realize that the voice in your head isn't you—it's simply noise.

The sequence is to notice the distortion, create some space using whatever tools work for you, then move toward what you want. You don't have to change your entire life. Change your relationship to your thoughts, and your life changes automatically. As people age, they often say they have more peace because they've stopped caring about what others think. What they've done is loosen their grip on the stories their minds have been telling them for decades. The most powerful realization? These stories were never real to begin with.

Remember David Burns's three-column technique outlined in chapter 7? You write the disruptive thought in the first column, note the type of distortion it is in the second, and write a more rational thought in the third (which I consider an optional step). After the first two columns, you have already created awareness and separation. Reprogramming happens as you move forward with your day, having made space for more positive inputs. The three-column method is a powerful reprogramming tool and increases awareness about the stories we tell ourselves. By recognizing each distortion that feeds the story of our ego, the house of cards we call ego is gradually pulled apart. What's left? It's you.

Ingrained Patterns

Becoming aware of our ingrained patterns means understanding the unconscious programming that shapes our reactions before we even realize we're reacting. Most of what drives your daily reactions isn't actually happening today; it's an echo from your past. By definition, you'll never become aware of it. You can only ascertain it by your reaction to triggering events. Your brain is constantly comparing today's experiences with everything you've ever learned about pleasure and pain. When something triggers anxiety or frustration, you're not responding to what's happening in the moment—you're reacting to a memory of something similar that felt threatening before. Ask yourself, "Am I alive, or am I just surviving?" You're only truly alive when you're experiencing today for what it is, not through the filter of yesterday's fears.

Your brain is constantly changing, evaluating your relationship with your environment, and interpreting sensations produced by your body. This idea is known as the pattern theory of self (PTS).[8] So, you have two dynamic senses of self: (1) in relation to yourself, and (2) in relation to the outside world. Your sense of identity in relation to yourself refers to your interactions with your own sensory input; this is the experiential aspect of self in your present reality. Your sense of self in relation to the outside world is narrative- or story-based; this is your social identity, establishing your place in the world. It can become rigid. There are typical patterns of interactivity between brain networks that create these two categories of self. It is not a fixed point.

PTS conceptualizes self not as a single unified entity but as a pattern of dynamically related factors unique to an individual. These include bodily, affective, behavioral, cognitive, narrative, and social processes that act in nonlinear, dynamic ways over varying time scales. Disruption of your unique functional patterns leads to mental rigidity, and, at some tipping point, it becomes problematic. Defending an unconscious, rigid identity with conscious means is a primary core issue, creating obsessive thought patterns. As you continue to pursue a stronger ego identity for the reasons outlined in chapter 9, these dynamic interactions change and are broken, with increasing mental rigidity. There is no logical end point for using the conscious to battle the unconscious.

There are functional networks in the brain that are defined by patterns of synchronized activity. There are seven recognized major large-scale networks. Two of them are fundamental neural systems for self-processing: (1) The default mode network (DMN), which is associated with self-processing; and (2) a set of three task-positive networks associated with your relationship to the world. These externally directed networks are the salience network (enhanced present-moment awareness), the control network (improved cognitive function), and the somatosensory network (embodied awareness).[9] Consider these three as a unit.

Disruptive mental rigidity results from the DMN being stuck in excessive self-referential processing and an inability to disengage from a self-focused narrative. This causes you to be caught in past- and future-oriented thinking, along with persistent rumination and worry.[10] This is one of the reasons that continually working on self-improvement is of limited value. You are not only stirring the same pot, but the pot is being stirred on its own. It is why bringing new data into your nervous system is essential for healing.

The other set of outward-facing task-positive networks is constantly counterbalancing your inward-focused DMN. It is essential to see how your actions based on how you feel work, or not.

Control usually switches smoothly between the internally focused DMN and the task-positive networks. Rigidity hampers this dynamic balance, leading to difficulty in quickly shifting between the internal DMN and external attention (task-positive). As a result, the DMN continues generating repetitive thoughts without properly comparing them with reality. Both networks become more embedded and stable; they are less responsive to each other, and cognitive interventions are less impactful. The DMN is like a clay pigeon thrower at a shooting range, launching thoughts without adequate control.

Later in this chapter, we will see how mindfulness-based interventions (MBIs) can increase the connectivity between these brain regions.

The Problem with Rehashing the Past

The mental health field often explores childhood experiences as if understanding one's past in great detail will somehow heal the person. While connecting with the roots of your emotional patterns can be an effective step toward healing, it's important to do so with awareness and in service to the present. True healing happens in a safe environment, not by reliving trauma. Your ability to find safety today does not depend on a response you had thirty years ago. Rehashing the past again and again strengthens those old neural circuits—precisely the opposite of what you want. What calming approach can you use now?

A Word About Mental Health Professionals

The support of a skilled and caring mental health professional can be incredibly valuable and is sometimes necessary. Experienced clinicians possess a lot of wisdom and can offer ongoing guidance and healing support. Modern trauma therapy and other forms of talk therapy often focus on helping you feel safe when experiencing intense emotions. Various psychotherapies frequently use calming modalities. Biofeedback allows a patient to see their bodily responses to interactions with the practitioner and other inputs. By watching the monitors hooked up to your body, you can train yourself to relax. Other calming tools include light touch chiropractic care, acupuncture, massage, and music. These can be used in the context of feeling unpleasant emotions as they arise.

Most mental health counselors understand their clients' issues and focus on guiding them out safely. Again, this book is not intended to be a substitute for traditional mental health care. These foundational concepts can help many people heal, but mental health experts help move people forward when they are stuck in the whirlpool of RUTs. I am a firm believer in mental health support. The reality is that insurance coverage is spotty at best. Psychologists who take health plans have limited access to benefits, and the services of health coaches and counselors are almost never covered. A major catch-22 is that the people who need these health resources the most often lack the financial resources to pay for them, since their ability to work is compromised. Our health insurance and workers' compensation systems are problematic and let too many people slip through the cracks.

This lack of access to mental health services has been a significant reason why I've spent so many years developing the

Dynamic Healing approach and writing books about the healing process. Modern medicine continues to overlook the data documenting the physiological nature of chronic pain and mental illness. There are concepts and strategies that anyone can start to use right now, with or without other professional supports.

In my clinical practice, patients often became upset when I suggested they see a psychologist because they felt I didn't believe them. "You're saying the pain is in my head." I always believed them, but I did not always know how to help.

Knowing what I know now, I would have recommended mental health support to almost every chronically ill patient who came to see me. It is challenging to put a life back together after chronic illness has torn it apart. Sometimes you need professionals to help break through the mental rigidity.

While I was in clinical practice, and now as I help people through my courses, I made a point of not talking to my patients or students about their personal problems. This is partly because I'm an MD, not a licensed mental health counselor, but it's also because I quickly realized that once someone started to share their troubles, we both got pulled into quicksand. Their pain was being unintentionally reinforced. This is why I adopted the approach of not discussing their pain or negativity more than strictly necessary. Most of the time, after a careful evaluation, I would check in with them briefly and then focus on solutions. It was much more effective to help them flip the switch and move on.

Analyzing the past to hunt down all the reasons you are triggered today creates a trauma story that becomes an anchor for your victimhood. Awareness allows you to connect with unpleasant emotions and memories in order to recognize that they are part of your past programming. Fully understanding your past and linking every present trigger to a past event is not necessary. Who really knows what the exact trigger for an emotional reaction might be today?

MINDFULNESS

Mindfulness-based interventions have been shown to disrupt cognitive fusion and mental rigidity.[11] While mindfulness offers a direct and effective approach to healing, chronic pain is complex, and mindfulness alone is just the beginning. It is essential to build a safety net as your defenses lower. The safety net is created by having the tools to regulate your body's physiology and occupy any color (emotional state) in the circle of life. You possess confidence from being connected to your reality through awareness.

An extensive prospective study conducted in England indicated that teaching mindfulness in middle schools offers limited benefits and can present challenges for students with emotional issues.[12] There is about a 10 percent likelihood of decompensation in another study.[13] If rigidity acts as a shield against raw anxiety, breaking through it without guidance on managing vulnerability is likely to cause difficulties. "The inverted U" describes this phenomenon. Usually, there is an initial period of significant benefit followed by a plateau or even a decline. Unfortunately, people often overestimate the benefits of mindfulness interventions and fail to address possible downsides adequately. Part of the problem is that follow-up periods are often too short to identify complications. Mindfulness is a helpful—and for some, essential—component of improving mental flexibility, but it should be one component of a comprehensive treatment plan. You need to learn tools to feel safe while working toward greater flexibility.

So, how do you handle ingrained patterns if you can't eliminate them and digging up the past only reinforces them? Notice them as they appear today. Anytime you feel anxious or frustrated, you're experiencing a preprogrammed response. That's all you need to understand. You don't need to know why. Linking every pattern to a specific event in the past is often just guesswork, and it wastes energy you could be using to engage with your life today.

Each time you have a strong reaction, it is part of a deeply embedded pattern. Become aware of it, separate from it, and calm your physiology using whatever tools work for you, then choose the direction you want to go. Since these patterns aren't based on current reality, there's nothing to fix—just notice, detach, and redirect. Engaging with them keeps them alive. Separating from them with awareness allows them to fade naturally. Remember, safety comes first.

Imagine a bamboo grove that bends with the wind and then rises again. Every "fail" shapes your success on the healing journey and is actually a chance to practice your skills, so strive for flexibility at every step. Trying to stick to a specific mindset or emotional state can be counterproductive. In *Antifragile: Things That Gain from Disorder*, Nassim Nicholas Taleb describes three states of existence: fragile, resilient, and antifragile.[14] Antifragile only exists in living organisms, which grow stronger in response to stress. Everything else, including resilience, eventually breaks. The goal isn't to become someone else; it's to intentionally choose and develop new patterns of thought and behavior that will lead to who you will become next—starting today.

These four types of awareness—sensory, emotional, judgmental storytelling, and ingrained patterns—aren't separate practices but facets of a single diamond. Environmental awareness grounds you in the present moment through external anchors. Emotional awareness helps you recognize and manage your internal states. Awareness of storytelling reveals the stories that create unnecessary judgment and suffering. Awareness of ingrained patterns shows when you're reacting to the past instead of responding to the present. Together, they form a comprehensive practice that addresses every way we disconnect from the present moment.

Summary

Healing happens by letting go of pain, anxiety, anger, and RUTs instead of trying to control them. We gain strength through vulnerability, not defensiveness; we find power in choosing to feel rather than suppress emotions; and we can make any challenge manageable when we approach it with awareness rather than reactive force. Awareness isn't just another tool—it's the foundation of healing. What you fight against becomes stronger; what you observe with awareness begins to change. In the end, all the strategies in this book boil down to different forms of awareness. With patience and persistence, connect to the present moment again and again, and your body will take care of the rest.

"All You Need Is Love" by the Beatles is a beautiful, simple song that delivers a powerful message: Love is at the heart of a meaningful life. Love and awareness are essentially the same. Just as the Beatles recognized that love transcends all boundaries, awareness surpasses all the complexities of healing. Love and awareness are the same state of being, healing and connecting every aspect of our physiology. "All you need is awareness, awareness . . . awareness is all you need."

CHAPTER 12

Be a Professional at Living Your Life

Success is peace of mind which is a direct result of self-satisfaction in knowing you made the effort to become the best you are capable of becoming.

—JOHN WOODEN, *Wooden: A Lifetime of Observations and Reflections On and Off the Court*

My goal in writing this book has been to create a shift in your outlook on life, enabling you to spend more time feeling safe. I am confident that you can transcend pain, anxiety, anger, and RUTs. However, this requires you to become a professional at living life—so you can skillfully navigate adversity and nurture joy.

Reading this book (or any other) alone won't decrease your RUTs. Can you learn to play the piano just by reading a book? Could I perform spine surgery simply by listening to lectures or watching it be done? All performances require coaching, learning, and practice, and life is a performance on the world's stage.

You can think of this book as an introductory training manual to help you frame your thinking and decide which resources to pursue to become an expert at living your life. Instead of evaluating yourself or worrying about the outcome, focus on growing your skill set. As you discover what works and what doesn't, you can adjust your strategies or refine your skills. This means you are learning from both your mistakes and your successes. Awareness is at the core of this process.

Life is a high-stakes game. We must fight daily to stay alive, let alone thrive. You might say, "I don't feel like I am fighting to stay alive." You are lucky because, for so much of life on this earth, there is no other choice.

You have the option of asking yourself, "Am I really alive? Is this living or just reacting?" And then, if you don't like the answer, you can do something about it. Instead of thinking about your life in terms of years, consider how much time you spend fully present in the here and now.

Seek Safety, Not Pleasure or Happiness

When asked what we want out of life, many of us would say, "I want to be happy." But what does that mean? How do we achieve that? No one is entitled to a happy life. It won't be handed to us. We often mistake happiness for pleasure, which is a transient state—part of our survival physiology whose counterpart is pain. Yet, the constant pursuit of pleasure, which requires repeatedly activating the dopamine circuit, often leads to greater pain and unhappiness. A hedonistic lifestyle makes inflammatory cells more aggressive. Every effort to avoid pain can become addictive. Addictions stem from the need to escape constant anxiety.

The marketing world targets these pain and pleasure receptors, generating huge demand by advertising images of happiness that most of us can't attain. This triggers envy, FOMO, and schadenfreude. The quickest way to activate pleasure circuits is through schadenfreude. The consumer market—everything from beauty products to home entertainment—is aware of this and utilizes neuroscience to latch on to our brains. Don't be fooled.

Stop seeking more power, control, and pleasure. A far more sustainable goal than happiness is safety. In safety physiology, you feel connected, confident, and content in the face of life's ups and downs. There is no other place you need to go. When you feel safe, you don't have to defend yourself or act out. You are grounded in the awareness of who you are, what you need, what you want, and what you can accomplish. Instead of "be all that you can be," just be. In this state, the body heals, and you are free to navigate your life in any direction you choose.

What is surprising is how many people in affluent societies who have plenty of resources are also miserable. Anxiety, anger, and RUTs lack sociological boundaries. We are all vulnerable to life's uncertainties, and luck also plays a role. We all share the same physiology and evolutionary wiring. Life's challenges will never end, and RUTs will keep turning up. But with the necessary skills, we can choose how we respond to them and navigate to safety.

The Social Determinants of Health

I want to acknowledge the many people who live in challenging, unsafe circumstances. I don't want to minimize their suffering or their struggles to find safety. Far too many people are living in war zones, experiencing famine, living in poverty, imprisoned, homeless, or otherwise trapped in circumstances that offer few opportunities to thrive. Part of being human means doing what we can to help one another, both individually and societally.

The social determinants of health are the nonmedical factors that influence health outcomes. Where we live, learn, work, and age, along with socioeconomic status and race, all have a tremendous influence on our health. They account for 80 percent of a person's health, while doctors influence about 20 percent.[1] Preventive public health efforts have never addressed the scope of our social issues. Environmental medicine addresses poverty, pollution, lack of opportunity, economic disparity, education, and a host of other issues. We tend to focus on symptoms rather than looking at patients in the context of their living circumstances. This part of our mandate as physicians has been overlooked. The incidence of diagnosable anxiety disorder is 100 percent if your income is less than $40,000 a year in the United States.[2] I believe it is possible to find peace of mind even in difficult circumstances, but it's more challenging.

Rising Above RUTs

Creating safety requires both skills and equipment. Consider these two types of flying: flying a kite and piloting a fighter jet. With a kite, you can reach great heights, but you have little control. Your decisions are limited to letting out or winding in the string. You're dependent on the weather and can't rise above it. Your equipment is fragile and no match for strong winds.

A fighter jet, on the other hand, can swiftly reach altitudes of 50,000 to 60,000 feet, surpassing even severe thunderstorms. You can smoothly conduct surveillance missions and land for refueling and maintenance. Both you and the aircraft can operate at maximum readiness when needed. If you're training to become a fighter pilot, you might start with flying a single-engine Cessna. Besides technical training, the primary measure of expertise is the number of hours flown. Nothing replaces time and practice. Don't expect to jump from a single-engine plane directly to a jet. Physical conditioning is also crucial; jet pilots must maintain excellent physical shape to handle the forces experienced during midair maneuvers.

You might say, "I could never be a jet pilot. How can I attain these advanced life skills?" Anyone can learn these skills, as long as you're open to learning and you make a commitment to practice. People often judge their progress by their pain levels or how often they experience RUTs, but this is a counterproductive way to think about it. You're focusing on your pain. Judging your abilities is a different matter. "What can I do? What's my current condition? Where can I improve? What are my strengths and weaknesses? Do I need guidance in a particular area? What are my blind spots?" You're not battling the storm; you're learning how to fly above it. The turbulence that used to define you and your world is now just weather. Climb through it to reach your flight level.

Being well trained with high-quality tools reduces your time on defense, so you can spend more time cruising. A fighter pilot only fights when necessary and when ordered to do so. Most of the time is spent on surveillance, patrol, or resting on the ground. Since RUTs don't really exist, you can fly right through them as they bounce off your jet.

The Performance Model

Consistency is the goal of any performance. The formula performance = skill − interference was developed by Timothy Gallwey, a Harvard-educated tennis player; he observed that his students often performed worse when he provided more technical instruction. They would overthink, tighten up, and lose their natural abilities.[3] This explained my struggle to develop a good golf game. Surgically analyzing every swing wasn't helpful.

In 2003, I returned to Seattle after spending four years in Sun Valley, Idaho. With more time in Sun Valley to play and practice, I took golf lessons but completely lost my swing. I went from shooting in the mid-80s to not coming close to breaking 100. Soon after returning to Seattle, I met David Elaimy, a golf pro who had played Division I golf for the University of Washington. Babs was also taking lessons, and from the start, he kept talking to me about my mindset in light of the performance = skill - interference formula. I kept telling him, "That is fine, but I just want a golf swing."

In 2006, my son, Nick, and his close friend, Holt, were struggling to compete in World Cup mogul skiing. It was clear that they both had the skills but lacked consistency. In October 2006, I flew them to Seattle to meet with David Elaimy. As he explained the performance formula, I finally understood his perspective for the first time. Holt went on to win the National Championship the following year, and Nick was ranked fifth in North America.

I realized that surgery is also a performance, so I engaged David as my coach. I truly enjoyed being a surgeon. Each case felt like a new performance, and I started each day in the operating room by introducing the patient to the team and encouraging everyone to share their thoughts about their roles. My technical complications decreased significantly.

David and I developed a training program that we used for workshops and to train my spine fellows. We recognized that, after many years of medical training, the fellows had a specific set of skills. However, few of them had been taught about performance principles. The first thing we asked was, "Which type of surgeon would you choose to work on you? Would you want an A-level surgeon, who is among the best in their field but is experiencing significant stress and occasional bad days? Or would you prefer a B-level surgeon who understands their limits and consistently does good work; and who would refer your case to someone else if it fell outside their expertise?" Naturally, everyone said they'd prefer to be operated on by a dependable B-level surgeon.

Consistency comes from continually improving skills and managing interferences. There are five types of interference: anxious, angry, distracted, complacent, and rushed. We introduced the awareness, intention, response (AIR) technique, which is a form of active meditation. I used this technique during surgery. The first step is to recognize when interference is occurring, identify it, and take a deep breath.

When I felt frustration, I might step away from the table. Then, I would visualize how I wanted to perform the next move, and respond accordingly. This AIR technique aligned with my 5-3-2 strategy (mentioned in chapter 3). I practiced this dozens of times per case until it became so ingrained in me that making safe moves became automatic. It also helped block out the many distracting thoughts that often arise during lengthy, stressful procedures. My mind quieted enough to complete an eight-hour case immersed in every move, with only a few disruptive thoughts throughout. Mindfully connecting with each move was much easier than fighting to concentrate. Awareness became the link to what was right in front of me.

Using this simple AIR technique, I was able to acknowledge the emotional interferences. Awareness created a safe space to feel, recenter, and move on with intention. This allowed me to visualize the anatomy in clear focus and perform a maneuver in a safe direction away from the spinal cord. Practicing environmental awareness—absorbing the sensations of each surgical step—became so embedded in my movements that to make an *unsafe* move, I would have had to make a conscious decision to do so. My safety buffer became quite wide. Self-judgment decreased and confidence grew as I focused on assessing my skills and making continuous improvements. Instead of fixating on a perfect performance and outcome, I connected with each moment, noticing less-than-ideal moves as they occurred and making midstream adjustments. I actively looked for them.

All of these performance principles can apply to how you live your life. Instead of monitoring your success, continually assess your skills and make corrections. Address minor issues to prevent larger problems. Each time you "fail" and keep moving forward, you are making progress. Practice awareness until it becomes habitual, and you will find yourself waking up to your own life. Don't force it; simply let it happen. Responding to reality is much easier than flailing at unseen adversaries. Notice how your mind quiets down.

Since sports are a meaningful part of my life, and they naturally illustrate many of the themes in this concluding chapter, they come up frequently in the following pages. If you are a sports lover, great. If you gravitate more toward the arts, like my wife, that's great, too. Keep in mind that any performative experience is relevant to the performance model.

Nick's Story

My son, Nick, is an exceptionally talented athlete who won the Junior Nationals in dual moguls for two consecutive years. He was on a promising path to the Olympic team. One day, while skiing in Sun Valley with four of his incredible (insane) skiing buddies, they ended their day by racing straight down the hill. Traveling close to sixty miles per hour, Nick's ski struck a small rock hidden in the snow. At that speed, even a minor obstacle can cause chaos. He flew approximately twenty to thirty feet forward, narrowly missing a tree, and landed on his left shoulder, which immediately dislocated. In that moment, he felt, for the first time, that he was going to die.

Until that incident, Nick had been fearless. However, when he returned to skiing the following season, he skied defensively. When you ski to avoid losing, it's impossible to win. Sound familiar? The next few years were tough, characterized by several injuries. After he ruptured a disc in his lower back, I encouraged him to let it all go and move on. As expected, he didn't listen to his father's advice and worked even harder. He was now twenty-nine.

Every December, the national qualifying event is called US Selections. The top two finishers earn guaranteed spots on the US ski team. In 2013, the two-day event was held in Winter Park, Colorado. There were two separate events, and it was the combined score of the two events that determined if Nick would qualify for the team, and possibly the Olympics. On the first day of competition, he qualified thirteenth out of seventy-five skiers. This advanced him to the finals, where he finished sixth, keeping him in contention for a top-two finish. On the second day, he qualified eleventh with an impressive run. However, anything less than first or second place in the final would not be enough. He did it! He skied the run of his life. In the final run, he missed first place by a single one-hundredth of a point.

I asked him how he had raised his skiing level to nearly winning the event. That's when he told me he had been doing a lot of expressive writing, and then immediately destroying it. I was both surprised and pleased that my son had taken his father's advice to heart. He had significantly increased his writing during competition week and was also using visualization techniques.

Before his final run, Nick confronted his deep fears of failing under pressure. At the starting gate, he grabbed his ski pole and wrote the word *fail* in the snow, then used his skis to smash it. He went on to ski the run of his life.

You can't outrun fear, nor can you conquer it; you must walk straight through it. Fully engaging with every part of an experience in the moment, including feeling the fear, helps to set aside the fear.

Holt's Story

In March 2007, our family watched the US National Championship in moguls. Nick had a tough day and didn't make it to the finals. He had been encouraged to try a trick he hadn't mastered and couldn't land during the competition. His friend Holt, meanwhile, had a great run and qualified in second place, while the top skier on the US ski team finished third. The top twelve skiers out of fifty advanced to a second run, with no points carrying over from the first.

It was around four in the afternoon when the final run was winding down. The sun hung low. The flat light caused by low clouds made it much more challenging to see the contours of the moguls. The top US ski team skier completed his run almost flawlessly, earning an impressive 27.2 out of a possible 30. Typically, a score above 26.5 has a strong chance of winning. Holt was the next skier. We all wished him the best, hoping he would have a solid run and possibly finish second or third. He took his turn and scored a 27.6, winning the US Championship. We were ecstatic and stunned. It was an incredible run under any circumstances, but nearly impossible to achieve under that kind of pressure.

How did Holt pull it off? At that point, I couldn't grasp how visualization worked, or how it differed from positive thinking. I spent the next day picking Holt's brain, asking him how he had performed so well under those circumstances. Here's what he told me.

First, he acknowledged the intense anxiety associated with the high-stakes competition. He felt anxious, knowing he had to beat a high score. Instead of suppressing his anxiety, he embraced it. Then, he focused on the feeling of the breeze on his face and the tips of his skis sliding over the snow. When his mind drifted to the thought of failure, he brought his attention back to the sensations around him. In doing so, he detached himself from his negative thoughts. Next, he visualized the first few turns, then he skied his run. He had also practiced these mindfulness techniques throughout the entire season.

Holt said that, in the past, his strategy had been to suppress negative thoughts and emotions by trying to hype himself up. This method was considered a form of positive thinking. "Don't worry about the other skier's score." "Don't be nervous." "I can do it." However, the energy used to suppress negative feelings would have detracted from the focus and energy needed to perform. This time, he chose alternative neurological pathways that were essential for maximizing his performance.

Inadvertently, Holt used the sequence of awareness, separation, and reprogramming. Focusing on the previous skier's score increased his anxiety. He faced his fears and distanced himself from them through awareness. He used active meditation and visualization as tools to reprogram his thoughts. As he felt the breeze and listened to the sound of the snow beneath his skis, he became fully present in the moment. Reprogramming through visualization is a powerful method; by playing out the event vividly in your mind, it crowds out any other program. Mentally experiencing every small detail, from start to finish, kept him locked in.

The power of visualization was shown in a study with volunteers learning to play the piano.[4] Researchers divided the volunteers into two groups and asked them to learn a simple scale. One group used a real piano, while the other visualized themselves playing the scale. When tested on their ability to perform the scale, the results of both groups were the same. The researchers repeated the experiment with basketball players. One group practiced shooting free throws, and another group visualized them. The visualization group improved almost as much as the group that practiced physically.[5]

Visualization is used as a therapeutic tool for chronic physical pain and mental pain as well. Negative self-beliefs are problematic for many people, particularly those stemming from disturbing experiences, especially if they are prolonged. Imagery Rescripting (ImRs) involves the integration of positive or neutral imagery and corrective information into images to facilitate emotional processing, reduce imagery intrusions, and restructure underlying schema.[6] Variations include visualizing past traumas and then visualizing safer outcomes. Other techniques concentrate more on visualizing pleasant outcomes to help people address worry.[7] Multiple ongoing studies are looking at the role of visualization in treating chronic disorders. The emergence of virtual reality has created numerous promising possibilities. Visual imagery, whether self-directed or using virtual reality, focuses on providing relaxing visual input combined with music.[8] It generally has a significant positive effect on mood and pain. However, it should be used in the context of addressing all the factors affecting your pain.

Letting Go of the Outcome

I use sports performances as examples, but any performance you participate in is relevant. When you fixate on the outcome, you become less connected to the present moment, which can hurt your performance.

When golfers have the yips, it means they are suddenly missing short, easy putts and the harder they try, the worse it gets. Even top professionals experience this phenomenon. A kicker with an almost perfect record misses a relatively simple field goal, leading to the loss of a game or even a championship. A singer feels anxious and worried about making mistakes, which leads to a poor performance. Almost any task can suddenly seem impossible under pressure. Where does this pressure come from? It's still the same task: a makeable putt, a field goal, or a song you've sung hundreds of times. Why would the situation make a difference? It doesn't have to.

Letting go of the outcome occurs naturally when you fully connect to the present moment. This is especially true for managing RUTs and chronic pain. If you try to fight or eliminate them, you will only end up reinforcing them and letting them control the situation. "The best way out is through" is an age-old concept that Robert Frost is widely credited for popularizing in modern times.[9]

What are your life goals? Where are you heading? The only thing that will improve the quality of your life is connecting to the present moment you're in—including this one, while you're reading this sentence. That is all. Focus on developing the skills and awareness to do this. Instead of worrying about where you need to go, you can find yourself exactly where you need to be. These ideas are not new; they have been recognized for thousands of years, especially in Eastern philosophy. In the hurry and noise of times, much of this wisdom has been ignored. There are many ways to cultivate awareness and rewire your brain. I have laid out what has worked the most consistently for me, my patients, and participants in my courses and workshops. Find what works for you.

If it helps to see your life as a performance, or a series of them, the key is to focus on performing to the best of your ability, whether you win or lose. Winning or losing in any context is temporary, and winning won't compensate for the misery you cause yourself every other moment of your life. Learn how to connect with and appreciate each moment for what it presents—whether it's peace or excitement, pain or pleasure, or an opportunity to practice your life navigation skills.

The Talent Code

I mentioned Daniel Coyle's *The Talent Code* in chapter 4 to describe how we become geniuses at feeling pain. We can apply the same concepts to becoming skilled self-healers. I recommend reading Coyle's informative and entertaining book to learn how our brains assimilate new information. The author traveled the world, gathering insights from elite athletes and performers to understand how genius evolves. He found that it is rarely an inherent trait. Through numerous conversations, Coyle identified three core concepts:

1. deep learning
2. master coaching
3. ignition (obsessive repetition)

Deep Learning

Deep learning involves reprocessing new information in your mind to make it easily retrievable. Researchers have conducted many studies on deliberate learning, which they define as engaging in structured activities specifically designed to improve performance in a particular area.[10] Coyle states that deep learning strategies can increase learning by 500 to 600 percent, based on his observations of performance academies and other talent hot spots. His book focused on the highest-level performers. Still, his findings offer practical takeaways for all of us.

The deepest learning occurs when you correct your mistakes, which means you must take risks. Many people suffering from RUTs become risk-averse and avoid scenarios that might stir them up. Then, the avoidance becomes its own stress. If this sounds like you, it's important to focus on calming skills rather than ignoring or fighting your thoughts. This will create space for deeper learning.

Interestingly, video games are designed to promote deep learning. Dr. Steve Cole, a UCLA genomics professor, spent ten years creating video games. He pointed out that most of the time, players lose, and then they have to repeat the game to reach their previous point or sometimes start over. Although players enjoy winning, they are more driven by the challenge of failing and learning from it. He told me, "The reprogramming is separating the player from the play cycle and realizing that even if the play cycle doesn't 'succeed' in completing the game, it still succeeds in helping the player grow."[11] It turns out that the human brain is addicted to growth, and video game design taps into this fundamental instinct. Players become stronger, wiser, smarter, and more diversified, in the sense of discovering multiple routes to reach their goals. Each "failure cycle" is actually a learning cycle—an exercise cycle that makes players wiser and more adept.

Learning from failure is essential for advanced learning in any endeavor. We all use this approach to some degree, often without realizing it. If we want to learn how to paint, we might study techniques, color, and form—and then paint many amateur compositions before the elements start to cohere in a more satisfying way.

You want to "fail" in a safe manner. Consider complex flight simulators where young pilots make mistakes during their learning curve that would be fatal in real life. These drills often expose pilots to "emergencies" so they can develop their reflexes. Safety drills occur in many domains. Coaches in sports and other performance arts hold a debriefing after each performance to analyze mistakes in the name of improving future performances. You can do the same with how you're navigating your life with RUTs, pain, or other stressors. What is working and what is not? If you keep bouncing from treatment to treatment without understanding your coping skills, how can you improve your processing expertise—and most importantly, how can you nurture the life you want? All of this happens through trial, error, and thoughtful analysis.

Many of us took notes in class and memorized them. For example, one of my medical school classmates read through his notes only once. However, he would look at a page and not move on until he could repeat most of it back to himself or write it down. He finished third in my class. This contrasts with another college buddy who would read for hours and not retain the material. I would memorize for twenty minutes and then lie down to nap for ten, repeating this process multiple times. I also rearranged the material according to my internal mental grid as I gathered new information. I scanned for what I had missed and made sure I understood it. When it comes to learning, get creative, and don't be afraid to fail.

Master Coaching

Guidance from a master coach can ensure that you are practicing specific tools and techniques accurately. Everyone knows the saying "practice makes perfect." But what if you are practicing the wrong techniques or doing the right ones incorrectly? You could develop bad habits. Often, it requires an outside observer to notice small details and keep your repetitions within a careful, constructive range.

Similarly, help from a mental health professional can be beneficial and sometimes crucial, as you learn to navigate your emotional states and shift away from reactive threat physiology toward safety. The goal is to feel safe, whether you are connecting with your past or managing your emotions today. Coaching of any kind also offers valuable support. It's common to feel socially isolated during intense training, and caring human interactions with a trusted coach can be very restorative.

Ignition

Ignition refers to being so passionate and motivated about what you're doing that you engage in endless repetitions. Outside motivation can push you, but it cannot match your internal drive. Many of us remember being prodded by our parents to practice a musical instrument. They may have employed various strategies to motivate us to play. Consider a kid who can't put the guitar down and plays with a vengeance. Jimi Hendrix was known for carrying his guitar with him almost everywhere. Friends, bandmates, and anyone who knew him consistently reported that his guitar was like an extension of him; he'd take it with him at parties, to hotel rooms, backstage, and even just walking around. He was constantly playing, experimenting, and practicing.

Think about something you've learned well and that brings you fulfillment, whether it's your job, an artistic hobby, a musical instrument, a sport, or a new language. How many hours, days, and years have you invested in consistent practice to achieve a high level of performance? What is often referred to as "muscle memory" is neurological memory, formed from circuits etched repeatedly in the brain over time. You can bring similar passion and energy to healing and living a better life.

Dr. Bernie Siegel and Self-Induced Healing

Dr. Bernie Siegel is a renowned pediatric general surgeon who recognized the importance of human connection early in his career. His ideas gained widespread recognition with the publication of his book *Love, Medicine & Miracles* in 1986.[12] It remains a foundational work in the field of mind-body medicine. He also founded and led an exceptional cancer survivors' group with Dr. Brenda Stockdale serving as its director.

I have known Dr. Siegel for over a decade. He participated in one of my workshops at the Omega Institute. I have always been fascinated by people who survive terminal cancer. He has shared many captivating stories with me, but I struggled to understand how, against all odds, those terminal cancer survivors survived. I asked him and Dr. Stockdale to present the data to our informal scientific study group. Just before the meeting, I asked Dr. Siegel again about those exceptional patients who experienced spontaneous healing. He had heard me ask this question so many times that, in a somewhat frustrated voice, he said, "This is not spontaneous healing. It is self-induced healing." Then he said the key is to induce a state of safety.

I was a bit surprised. I hadn't heard him talk about self-induced healing or safety before. As he and Dr. Stockdale explained the concepts, I realized how similar they were to treating chronic pain. Cancer is highly linked to sustained threat responses, just like any ongoing mental or physical illness. Self-induced deep healing can also be seen as a way of creating self-induced safety.

One of Dr. Siegel's main points was that survivors stopped looking for answers and started living life on their terms. They made significant changes in lifestyle, finances, careers, and relationships. They understood they had limited time, so they committed to living it fully. Dr. Siegel said, "They were so busy living, they forgot to die." Don't just read about healing—start healing right now.

In the C-quence of healing, the ground represents your entire past. It is your source of learning and future growth. As you learn to acknowledge the darkest aspects of your past without reacting, your root system will grow stronger, branching out with a deep awareness of the patterns that are playing out today.

You are shifting from relying on external circumstances to heal toward strengthening your internal locus of control. You can gather data, talk to experts, and take in cues from your environment, but only you can decide what healing approach is best for you. Only you know what it feels like to be in your body—and how your thoughts and emotions affect you. Resolve to be an active participant in your healing process, rather than passively waiting for someone or something to fix your problems.

Find your ignition: What inspires and motivates you to pursue a better quality of life? Any world-class performer will tell you that no one but themselves can motivate them to practice as hard as they do. Ideally, excitement gives way to a playful approach, with a shift toward creativity. Most of us are already experts at experiencing pain. How can we employ deep learning, master coaching, and ignition to become equally skilled at "self-induced healing"—and at navigating life's challenges with awareness and creativity?

What Are Your Expectations?

Sit down, take a deep breath, and think about what you truly want. You might say that your goal is to be free from pain and RUTs forever. But how will you achieve that? Pain—whether mental or physical—is an ingrained memory that deepens over time. Those pain circuits won't magically disappear. Healing is not a linear journey.

I have had many patients who did remarkably well for a few months and were thrilled about their progress as the pain lifted. I regularly warned them that they would occasionally experience relapses, and these could be worse because the contrast would be more noticeable. Inevitably, even with my warnings, they would become very upset when the pain came back again. When stress reaches a certain point, you'll return to pain. That's what your body is supposed to do. I reminded them that they now had strategies to calm down and get back to healing. These conversations led to a metaphor about Major League Baseball, offering valuable insights about healing.

Major League Baseball

Think of your life journey as becoming a Major League Baseball player. You are the hitter, and life is the pitcher. The pitcher isn't your friend, nor is life, which throws every type of pitch at different speeds—fastball, curve, slider, sinker, and changeup. It can be delivered overhand, sidearm, or even underhand. It's almost miraculous when a human hits the ball. Some pitchers cheat by altering the surface of the ball with dirt, Vaseline, scratches, or spit. The ball moves so fast and with spin that the small irregularities on the surface change the dynamics and exaggerate the movement. It is actually dangerous for the hitter and catcher.

Baseball is considered one of the most intense and stressful sports, involving both individual contributions and team collaboration. It contrasts with sports like basketball or soccer, where effective teamwork through passing, defense, and strategy is just as vital. Individual mistakes in these other sports are less noticeable and typically have a minor impact on the final result. In baseball, however, both heroic acts and mistakes are highlighted. A single error or strikeout can decide the game or even a whole season. Remember that even the best players make outs most of the time.

Now let's consider the game of life. Like MLB players, people who are struggling to heal from pain have good days and bad days, with varying batting averages. You might say, "I don't know anything about baseball, and I don't want to." Guess what? You are in the game, regardless. Life keeps coming at us, and while we sometimes do well, often we don't. That isn't failure; it's just life. We are rarely taught the basic skills to effectively handle adversity, regulate our body's chemistry, and nurture joy. We are thrown into life, doing our best to survive. Our parents, teachers, peers, and society share their examples of how to live, but how

Practice, Practice, Practice

It takes years of repetition to develop a disciplined eye for "your pitch," to have the patience to walk (especially with two strikes), to have a consistently reproducible swing, and to maintain excellent physical condition. The ball takes about 0.4 second to reach the plate, and the batter has roughly 0.15 second to decide whether to swing. You must train your brain to recognize not just a ball in the strike zone but also one you can hit. You can't think about it; it requires tens of thousands of swings to master that skill. Hitting an MLB pitch is one of the most complex skills in sports.

Guess what? Processing stress is even more difficult. It will take a lot of practice to get from Little League to the majors. Initially, you will have limited skills, but it's essential to be kind to yourself no matter how you're doing at the plate. Many people initiate the healing process and experience improvement quickly. Then, they might be triggered, or severe stress could cause everything to fall apart. The tendency is to get angry and catastrophize that they've failed and won't be able to get back on their feet. The sooner they can accept that this is the nature of the game, that life just keeps throwing pitches, the more quickly they can adapt.

As you advance your skills, you'll encounter fewer triggers and spend less time in the hole. You can't avoid triggers, but they won't necessarily overpower you. Once you feel relief, the temptation might be to stop learning and practicing, but once you escape the abyss and make your first steps into the light, why would you stop there? With practice, practice, practice, you will master the calming and creative skills you need to feel safe and build the life you want.

many of them learned practical self-regulating skills? Where is the master coaching for the game of life? Is it any wonder that there is so much suffering and social chaos?

Summary

How long and hard do you want to fight your imaginary foes—your anxiety, anger, and RUTs—before your fuel tank runs empty and you crash? It is time to start treating your life like the most important job you'll ever have. It's time to learn to fly your jet. You might say, "I don't have a jet, and where would I find one?" You already have the most advanced model—your body. It has far more capacity to carry you anywhere you want and to defend you well. And unlike a jet, it will repair itself if you let it.

The only person who can guide this aircraft is you. You will need to make decisions based on the weather. Would you fly into the middle of a hurricane? What if the wings ice up? Do you know how to use the instruments to land in poor visibility? What if you are on a mission and in a dogfight? Do you have the skills to meet the challenge? Life can get rough, but you can learn how to fly through turbulence and reach blue skies.

Leave your old programming behind. Become a professional at living your life. The possibilities are endless.

Epilogue

We can make ourselves miserable or we can make ourselves strong. The amount of effort is the same.

—PEMA CHÖDRÖN, *When Things Fall Apart*

My panic attack on the Seattle bridge in 1990 didn't happen out of the blue. It started one day during my first few months of ninth grade when I metaphorically shut the door on my life and created a new identity.

My family life was chaotic and abusive. Without proper parental guidance and stability, I lacked confidence and was always seeking approval, looking for any sign that I was okay. The words *not good enough* carved themselves into my mind and became my internal compass. My father kept changing jobs, so by the time I was eighteen, we had lived in twelve different houses. Whenever I felt a sense of community, my family would move again. Seventh grade in Santa Cruz, California, was the first year I made some good friends. Just as I was enjoying myself, we moved to Bakersfield, and I had to start over in eighth grade. I had some nice friends, but I needed approval badly and worried that no one wanted to listen to me, which is why I spoke quickly, mumbled, and stuttered. The next summer, we moved to Napa. I felt overwhelmed.

In Napa, I started spending time at my friends' houses. Their home lives were strikingly different than mine. I remember the exact moment I mentally closed the door on my past and decided to forge a new identity. I didn't just close the door; I slammed it shut and set out on my own. Now I realize I dissociated.

I was good at it. I spent little time with my family and a lot of time with friends. I was obsessively busy. One year, I took twenty-one college credit hours in a quarter, played intramural sports, socialized, earned nearly straight A's, and worked construction five to ten hours a week.

What I didn't do was sleep much. I was energized by my new life and having a great time. I graduated magna cum laude from college, earned Alpha Omega Alpha Honors in medical school, got accepted into a competitive orthopedic residency, and trained at one of the top spinal deformity fellowships in the world. Stress? What stress? The "not good enough" voice was still there but harder to hear. No problem. I saw it as the key to my success.

In the winter of 1990, I was skiing in Utah with my six-year-old son in six inches of fresh snow. The skiing couldn't have been better, and I was sharing this experience with my son. I realized I had achieved everything I thought I needed to be happy, and I had followed the rules. But I couldn't have been more miserable. Furthermore, I had no idea what else to do, and I was getting tired. My ears were ringing loudly from tinnitus, skin rashes appeared randomly all over my body, my migraines worsened, and both feet burned. Also, my RUTs became more noticeable. But no, I didn't feel anxious, and I was definitely not angry.

About a month after that ski trip, while driving across the Seattle bridge, the lid blew off the pressure cooker I had locked into place in ninth grade. It exploded sky-high. I developed crippling anxiety and ongoing panic attacks, and no one could tell me what had happened or why. My close friends and I were stunned. They saw me as extremely confident and invincible. So did I.

I conducted a relentless search to understand what had happened. By 1997, my RUTs were severe. For the next seven years, I did everything possible just to get through each day. Relief only came when I was focused on performing surgery or in the clinic. Free time was a nightmare.

My New Perspective

What do I know now, thirty-five years later? My intense drive to build a strong ego was a defensive act, and the identity I proudly displayed was merely a façade. I crafted an image of who I wanted to be and how I wanted others to see me. But instead of being grounded in my core values, I was running from my pain. No one could have done it better. I was battling anxiety, anger, and imaginary threats—all of which were my friends and protectors. I was creating enemies out of nothing but my thoughts. At the mercy of my own harsh inner critic, there was no way I could win.

Humans are the most intelligent mammal species when we are using our highest thinking brains. However, we are hardly intelligent when reactive and angry. We are the only species that inflicts pain on our own kind, not for survival, but simply because we have different ideas. Other animals fight to stay alive; we fight over religion, politics, and race, and destroy each other over thoughts that have no physical substance. Our sapiocortex, which creates these abstract ideas, stops functioning optimally when it is needed to solve the problems it has caused.

Rodney King was a Black man who was severely beaten by police after refusing to pull over for speeding. At least twenty police officers watched without intervening as he sustained broken bones, a skull fracture, and brain damage. The officers' acquittal by a largely white jury sparked six days of rioting in Los Angeles. On the third day of the riots, King made a well-known plea on television: "People, I just want to say, can we all get along? Can we get along? Can we stop making it horrible for the older people and the kids?"[1]

The answer is yes, we can find peace, if we learn how to break through our defensive egos and connect to the PFC just behind our forehead. This region of our brain holds limitless creativity and problem-solving potential. Fortunately, modern neuroscience has enabled us to explore how the brain works and discover better ways to access it.

The first step is learning to feel safe. That means being kind to ourselves and others, regardless of how we feel. We can cultivate kindness, which arises from awareness. This is not a trivial suggestion. This changes the body's chemistry. Deep healing occurs as we nurture safety and bring the sapiocortex fully back online. At a certain tipping point, as we use our higher thinking powers to heal and create new neural pathways, our physiology gains momentum along a positive trajectory, and there's no turning back.

Robert's Story

Robert emailed one day about his chronic lower back pain, which had been bothering him for over five years. He had read many books on mind-body healing, including *Back in Control*, but he was still experiencing some lingering symptoms. He was curious about what else he could try. I am not sure how the conversation shifted toward unwanted thoughts, but it quickly became clear that he was being overwhelmed by intense, intrusive thoughts.

Robert was a social worker living in the Northeast. In his mid-thirties, he had been working for the state for ten years, focusing on family issues and protective services. Anxiety had been a problem for him since his early teens, and intrusive thoughts became problematic in his early twenties. By his mid-twenties, they were affecting his quality of life, and he felt trapped, growing more desperate to escape. He read over a hundred self-help books on intrusive thoughts, underwent extensive counseling, took various medications, practiced meditation, and used thought-stopping techniques. His relentless quest to find a way out did not improve his symptoms; instead, they worsened. He became discouraged and depressed as hope faded. Somehow, he remained functional, and like me, no one around him could see how much he was suffering.

I told him I had helped many people overcome chronic physical pain, and that mental pain is often more crippling. I shared with him that RUTs were the worst part of my fifteen-year struggle in the abyss. I had escaped my relentless barrage of unwanted thoughts, and the occasional ones that arose weren't disruptive. He was interested in learning how to escape the same abyss that had trapped me. He engaged in the self-directed course I had assembled called The DOC Journey. As he learned the healing concepts, he noticed a marked improvement within the first three months. Over the following year, as he customized the healing framework to his own pace and needs, his intrusive thoughts resolved.

Robert told me, "The idea that intrusive thoughts are solvable is revolutionary." For years, he had read and heard about the poor prognosis for people like him. I had also read countless books on the subject and gotten the same impression. Imagine our excitement at the discovery that there is a way out.

This book grew from the seeds of Robert's story and mine. The clarity with which Robert has shared his healing journey with me has enabled me to write this book. It also grew from countless other success stories, only some of which made it onto these pages. I did not leave spine surgery to manage pain, but to follow a path of hope and discovery. Witnessing hundreds of people emerge from the depths of despair to thrive beyond their expectations has been incredibly inspiring.

Think of the energy you spend on fighting your negative thoughts. Imagine if, instead, you could redirect all that energy toward living your life, creatively and on your own terms. I am still amazed by how energized I feel now. Each day I am free of RUTs feels like a gift.

Going Forward

Thoughts become very real as they fuse with our identity. This is why hearing others express opposing ideas and beliefs can feel like a personal attack. Ruminations and rigidity are traits that cross almost every mental health diagnosis, and they are not being adequately addressed. Instead of connecting as a family of human beings, we are crashing our egos into one another and causing a lot of pain and misery. With a clearer understanding of what's happening on the physiological level when we routinely feel pain, anxiety, and anger, and are plagued by RUTs, we can devise effective solutions.

Many research centers around the world are generating deep insights with new technological advances. We can look into the cell and understand interactions we never knew existed. Elaborate physiological pathways are being discovered with potential therapeutic interventions. The roles of mitochondria and DNA are being further explored. Brain circuits are being mapped with greater accuracy. With AI, more collaboration is possible, and the next wave of learning will be powerful.

Many practitioners across all health fields are adopting these healing principles based on the physiology of chronic illness. Instead of seeing chronic disease as unsolvable, they are viewing it as highly treatable, while allowing patients to direct their own care. The public health implications of these physiological principles and healing tools are especially encouraging, since many of the resources needed for healing are now easily accessible. However, mainstream medicine is still lagging far behind the scientific wisdom. It is time to advocate for more public education and infrastructure.

Opportunities for societal change are most significant in school systems. The importance of play and healthy social interactions is gaining recognition, and programs are being introduced to teach social-emotional skills starting in elementary school. However, this is just the beginning of what needs to happen to create a larger societal shift.

As a human species, we need to start activating the highest functions of our brains. Let's stop spending our lives on guard and playing defense. Let's start creating the safe space we need to step out of our egos, stop reacting to imaginary threats, and become the creative directors of our own lives.

The world needs you to heal. That is your only responsibility. The ripple effects of your own healing journey will extend to your family, friends, colleagues, and community. You don't have to save the world—just yourself.

Acknowledgments

I could not have written any of my books without the help of Ray Bunnage, an expert in the tech world, a close friend, and someone who is dedicated to analyzing data to help make the world a better place. Many years ago, he observed that I was "energized by my patients." I hadn't thought about it much before, but he was right. I am constantly inspired not only by my patients' successes, but even more by their courage and commitment to healing in the face of significant challenges.

This phase of my journey began with a backyard conversation with my wife's tango teacher, David Orley Thompson, in 2019. I had tried to read Steve Porges's book, *The Polyvagal Theory*, but I did not understand its relevance to spine surgery. David was excited about it. I felt that if he could see its importance, so should I, so I took the book to Patagonia on a fishing trip and read it properly. I was blown away. Many concepts about chronic illness began to come together. This was just the beginning of a remarkable journey.

Hara Marano—editor at large at *Psychology Today*, and the person who provided me with Steve Porges's email address—has played a key role in shaping ideas.

Steve and his wife, Sue Carter, introduced me to a whole new world of evolutionary biology and neurophysiology. I truly appreciate their openness, knowledge, support, and friendship. Thanks to our informal study group, the connections and concepts that inform this book have expanded significantly.

I want to thank the members of our Dynamic Healing Discussion Group. They continue to share insights and support my ongoing efforts. I wish to acknowledge a few individuals in particular. I talk with DR Clawson more often than I do with my wife. He has a remarkable ability to think across disciplines and create new narratives. Les Aria has trained me in applying polyvagal principles to clinical care, and we enjoy learning together.

Members who have made significant foundational contributions to this repository include Bob Naviaux (mitochondria), Dick Gevirtz (autonomic nervous system regulation), Steve Cole (genomics and social factors affecting the immune system), Mel Pohl (addiction medicine), and Steve Overman (rheumatology). Back in 1990, Steve Overman told me, "Hey, Hanscom, it's the inflammation." Of course, from my surgical perspective, I didn't believe him. Jamie Pennebaker has supported me for many years, and his ability to listen and share his wisdom has been wonderful. Linda Stone has been insightful, clear, and instrumental in keeping the study group moving forward, and she has been a source of encouragement.

Les Kertay has spent hours with me reviewing the concepts in this book. I had thought the basic human drive is to avoid anxiety, but he made clear to me that our main need is to feel safe. Kari Briscoe has spent time with both of us and has been incredibly supportive of our efforts.

Many colleagues have contributed to my efforts: David Tauben taught me to listen; Jim Robinson challenged me; Jake Eagle added his perspective on A.W.E.; Bernie Siegel inspired me with his wisdom; Mark Tomski offered deep philosophical insights; Suzanne LaCrosse showed me the value of the doctor-patient relationship; Gordon Irving demonstrated the importance of a multidisciplinary approach; Geralyn Datz provided perspective on cognitive-behavioral therapy; David Cassius introduced me to a new world of soft tissue work; Mags Clark-Smith is remarkable in her somatic approach; Rod Oskouian set up an exceptional spine fellowship and demonstrated technical surgical expertise; Kendra Bloom helped many patients I thought had no chance of healing; and Marc Moisi took these concepts and created a thriving spine center.

Howard Schubiner introduced the foundational healing ideas in 2009 when he was a keynote speaker at one of my courses. His ongoing research and teaching efforts are impressive, as is his golf game (he destroys me on the course). Joel Konikow was my wingman for years. He was the pain physician I worked with most closely, and his patient care was magical. He taught me patience.

Doug Garland is a mentor and friend who introduced me to tall poppy syndrome (TPS), an important concept in this book. David Burns continues to inspire me with his boundless energy, and I would not have gotten through my years in the abyss without his book *Feeling Good.* Fred Luskin and I have lunch every month, and his insights on forgiveness and vulnerability have influenced my approach. Matt Lederman has taught me a lot about nonviolent communication, and his nutritional knowledge is impressive. Dave Sabey has inspired me for many decades, and he is mentoring a group of us on leadership. He was the one who showed me the value of maintaining a positive vision and nurturing joy. He also taught me never to waste a crisis or give up. Beth Grossman, my publicist for my previous books, has been encouraging me from the start. Bruce Lipton has shared his forward-thinking vision, and he is great to hang out with.

David Elaimy and I have shared a long journey. He was my coach for surgical performance and a source of great wisdom. I also want to thank Holt Haga, Daimon Bushi, and, especially, my son, Nick, for truly listening to David and me as we presented performance principles. They demonstrated them beautifully on the slopes, skiing at the highest level, despite facing a lot of adversity.

Every patient and individual who has engaged with these principles has inspired me. Some of them include Susi Casserd, Mark Owens, Sachit Egan, and Cole Brandenberger. I value their ongoing insights.

Chris and Michaele Dimock and I worked extremely hard together to create the DOC Journey course, which so many people have found healing. Justin Barker spent hours with me, helping me understand the importance of foundational awareness for healing. Joe Klemczewski and Jen Sounder met with me monthly for a year, allowing me to refine my message.

My friends Kevin and Patrice Auld and John Shervey have watched my saga from the beginning. I appreciate that they stuck with me.

My family never wavered in their support. My stepdaughter, Jasmine, and my wife, Babs, brought in the element of play. The workshops we held as a family were incredibly enjoyable. My brothers Alan and Bob formed a weekly writing club, and their rather clear (blunt) input helped shape this book.

Each member of my clinical and support staff has inspired and motivated me throughout my career. Their dedication to excellence and quality patient care is unmatched.

Leslie Meredith, my literary agent, believed in this project enough to take it on. I'm grateful to her for staying the course. Anna Bliss, my editor at Chelsea Green, has introduced me to a whole new level of writing. She had me basically rewrite this book and stayed with me every step of the way. She has a remarkable ability to pay attention to detail.

My A team has been the foundation of my efforts. Tom Masters, Mark Mendonca, Suzi Cairns, Marj Tabuclin, and my wife, Babs, have been a major force in advancing my efforts.

I want to thank my wife, especially, who saw something in me I couldn't see. My opening line on our first blind date was, "I have ADD and OCD, but I have worked through my anger issues." Then the roof caved in, and she stuck with me. Sue Carter has taught us about the healing power of oxytocin and human connection. I am a living testament to it.

I want to thank everyone who made a significant contribution to this work. Even the smallest comments and conversations have been impactful. It takes a village!

Glossary

adverse childhood experiences (ACE): A research construct from The ACE Study by Vincent Felitti and Robert Anda describing major categories of childhood trauma and their dose-dependent impacts on adult health, mental health, addiction, and social outcomes.

affective component: The emotional component of pain as opposed to somatosensory component.

agency: The sense of having control over one's actions and decisions that influence outcomes in one's life. It reflects the capacity to act intentionally, make choices, and initiate change, as opposed to passively reacting to circumstances or feeling powerless.

aggressive self-attack: Relentless self-criticism or internal verbal assault. This form of self-directed anger often manifests as harsh judgments, perfectionistic demands, and mental bullying, fueling chronic stress and pain circuits. The sapiocortex is hyperactive but not functioning optimally.

altruism: Behavior and attitudes based on concern for the well-being of others, often expressed through acts of kindness, support, or self-sacrifice. Research has shown it provides significant mental and physical health benefits.

amygdala: The core danger detector and alarm in the limbic system; triggers rapid fight-or-flight, anxiety, or anger responses.

anabolism: The repair and growth that occur in a state of safety physiology.

anger: A hyperactivated threat state that includes neurochemical changes such as elevated dopamine and endorphins. It is a powerful physiological response to a perceived or real threat, injustice, or frustration. It is not primarily a psychological issue.

anterior cingulate cortex (ACC): A frontal part of brain that is key for processing both physical and emotional pain, including experiences of social exclusion or envy; links pain perception and affect.

anxiety: A physiological state in which the body is mobilized in preparation for a threat. It simply says danger, even when it is not immediately present. It is not a psychological diagnosis.

appeasement vs. fawning: Appeasement is an unconscious, neurobiological survival strategy of genuine coregulation with a threat (in actual danger). Fawning is chronic people-pleasing, driven by the need to manage others' emotions long after real danger has passed.

automatic negative thoughts (ANTs): Term used by David Burns in *Feeling Good* to describe the mind's tendency to gravitate toward negative thoughts.

autonomic nervous system (ANS): Part of the nervous system that automatically controls and regulates involuntary body functions like heart rate, digestion, breathing, and blood pressure. It has two main divisions—the sympathetic and parasympathetic nervous systems—which work together to keep the internal environment of the body balanced and immediately able to respond to changes or stress.

awareness: The conscious recognition and observation of one's thoughts, feelings, bodily sensations, or environment—without judgment or reactivity. It allows for choice and separation from automatic, habitual patterns.

bidirectional loop: Repetitive unwanted thoughts and threat physiology maintain each other in a positive feedback cycle in which threats trigger intrusive thoughts, and those thoughts reinforce physiological threats, making both more entrenched.

C-reactive protein (CRP): A chemical marker that signals inflammation in the body. It can be elevated in infection, autoimmune disorders, and stress.

catabolism: Metabolic state under threat: fuel consumed for immediate energy.

central sensitization syndrome (CSS): A condition in which the nervous system is more sensitive to stress and the conduction velocity of the nerves increases.

chronic physical pain: The persistence of the memory of pain or the inability to extinguish the memory of pain evoked by an initial inciting injury. In other words, it is permanently embedded in your nervous system until you reprogram your neural circuitry.

cognitive-behavioral therapy: The branch of psychology that specifically addresses dysfunctional belief systems along with the associated behaviors.

cognitive dissonance: The discomfort created by conflicting beliefs or between beliefs and behavior, motivating maladaptive defense responses. Challenges to deeply held beliefs feel like personal attacks.

cognitive distortions: Systematic errors in thinking (e.g., labeling, "should" thinking, minimizing the positive, catastrophizing) that coalesce to form your ego. They fuel repetitive unwanted thoughts, anxiety, and anger.

cognitive fusion: The entanglement of identity with thoughts and beliefs, such that mental events become rigidly fused with the self and intensified by physiological threat.

compassion: A prosocial emotion involving empathy, understanding, and a desire to ease others' suffering. Self-compassion extends this caring attitude inward, counteracting self-criticism and perfectionism. It is the basis of compassion-focused therapy and is a powerful approach for resolving repetitive unwanted thoughts. Compassion is synonymous with love and awareness.

compulsive behaviors: Repetitive actions performed to reduce distress or discomfort—often in response to intrusive thoughts or anxiety—even when the behaviors are irrational or disruptive.

congenital indifference to pain: A disorder where babies are born without a protective pain system. Since they cannot protect themselves, they become quickly disfigured and typically live less than twenty years.

connection: Meaningful bonds or relationships with others, characterized by mutual trust, empathy, and attunement. Social connection is a biological necessity, decreasing inflammation and supporting mental and physical health. Oxytocin is a powerful social-bonding hormone that is anti-inflammatory. It is also a mediating hormone.

cranial nerves V, VII, VIII: Three of the twelve nerves that originate directly from the brain at its base. These are relevant to the calming effects of the vagus nerve (X). They are trigeminal (V), facial (VII), and auditory (VIII). Calming interventions include forehead touch and cold compresses, humming, singing, soothing music, and direct stimulation.

cranial nerve X (vagus nerve): Main parasympathetic "rest and digest" nerve that activates calming, anti-inflammatory, and healing processes and is key in safety signaling.

cytokines: Small proteins that act as signaling molecules between cells. Most active in the immune system.

pro-inflammatory (e.g., IL-6, TNF-alpha): upregulated in threat states, driving neuroinflammation, pain sensitization.

anti-inflammatory: active during safety, facilitating repair.

deep learning: Learning that occurs through meaningful, deliberate interaction with the material or situation, such as correcting mistakes and embracing "failure."

default mode network (DMN): Brain system responsible for idle, repetitive, self-referential thought; generates repetitive unwanted thoughts.

dissociating: The act of consciously or unconsciously separating from the past. This is an extreme form of thought suppression.

dorsolateral prefrontal cortex (dlPFC): The seat of working memory, abstract thought, and cognitive flexibility; most highly evolved and most susceptible to stress, inflammation, or threat states. Considered the core of the sapiocortex, which also includes several other high-functioning areas.

Dynamic Healing: A systems-based approach focusing on the interplay of input (stressors), processing (nervous system state), and output (behavior or symptoms); emphasizes shifting into safety physiology to break threat loops.

ego (identity): A constructed, often rigid sense of self, based on external validation and intended to protect against psychological pain and threats.

emotions: Feelings associated with the state of the body's physiology.

energy audit: The brain's ongoing prioritization of inputs based on perceived threat and resource depletion. When overwhelmed, threat signals are prioritized, worsening repetitive unwanted thoughts. This metaphor clarifies why stress and rumination become self-perpetuating and exhausting.

exteroception: Data collected from your environment through your body's sensors to be processed by the brain. It is the dynamic sum total of this input.

functional MRI (fMRI): A medical imaging technique whereby a labeled glucose (the brain's energy source) is injected into the body and MRI scans pick up which parts of the brain are active in relationship to specific activities and emotions.

heart rate variability: The variation in time intervals between heartbeats, serving as a marker for the adaptability of the autonomic nervous system and overall physiological resilience. More variability indicates higher safety physiology.

hippocampus: An area of the brain that is responsible for processing long- and short-term memory.

homeostasis: The body maintains a dynamic internal stability (temperature, pH, energy) based on every reaction having an almost equal opposite reaction. Homeostasis is the relative balance that is necessary for maintaining life.

insula: Region of the brain processing body sensations (interoception) and emotional pain; instigator of rigid, embodied beliefs, especially when stress is high.

insula-based beliefs: Beliefs formed during times of high threat or stress that feel physically real are stored in the insular cortex of the brain. The downregulated sapiocortex does not filter them, so they are rigid, emotionally charged, and resist logical change.

interoception: The summation of all sensory input to your body is called interoception. It is a complex system that allows you to feel your body's internal states.

ironic effect (paradoxical thought suppression): Attempts to suppress a thought paradoxically increase its frequency and intensity, as revealed by Daniel Wegner's "white bear" experiment.

limbic system: Central emotional circuitry that assumes control when threat is present, suppressing higher-level prefrontal cortex reasoning; includes the amygdala.

mental rigidity: Habitual, inflexible adherence to unhelpful cognitive, emotional, or behavioral patterns; resistant to change, and reinforced by threat physiology.

metacognition: Awareness of one's own thought processes, enabling perspective-taking and cognitive flexibility; impaired during intense cognitive fusion or stress. Capacity to think about thinking.

microglia: Brain's immune cells; when chronically activated by stress or threat, they generate neuroinflammation and contribute to cell axonal damage.

neuroception: A nonconscious process (in Polyvagal Theory) by which the nervous system filters cues from inside and outside the body to assess safety or danger.

neurological: Descriptive term for anything to do with the nervous system.

neuroplasticity: The brain's lifelong ability to rewire, shrink, expand, and adapt, for better or worse, in response to new experiences and practiced attention.

neurotransmitters

- **acetylcholine:** calming and excitatory neurotransmitter; activates muscles and calming in the parasympathetic nervous system.
- **dopamine:** motivation, pleasure, addiction, and drive—hyperactive in threat, craving, schadenfreude.
- **GABA:** main calming, inhibitory neurochemistry; increases with relaxation/safety.
- **glutamate:** main excitatory neurotransmitter; escalated in threat.
- **serotonin:** mood regulation, inhibition, restoration.

nucleus accumbens: Central dopaminergic "reward" region in the ventral striatum controlling habit reinforcement, pain relief via schadenfreude, and addiction behaviors.

orbitofrontal cortex (OFC): Region of the prefrontal cortex that regulates social behavior, impulse control, and adaptability. Stress undermines its function, reducing social flexibility.

parasympathetic nervous system (PNS): The division of the autonomic nervous system that promotes "rest and digest" functions by slowing heart rate, stimulating digestion, and supporting recovery after stress. It conserves energy, maintains basic bodily functions, and drives the body toward relaxation and safety.

pattern theory of self (PTS): Your brain is constantly changing and evaluating its relationship with your environment, and interpreting sensations produced by your body. PTS refers to a dynamic sense of self that is based on (1) your relationship to yourself, given present sensory inputs, and (2) your identity in relation to the outside world (ego). These two sets of circuits don't interact fluidly in mental rigidity.

peripheral nervous system (PNS): This refers to any part of the nervous system that is distal to (situated away from) the brain or spinal cord. It transmits input from the environment to the central nervous system.

physiology: The functions of living organisms.

Polyvagal Theory: A model of nervous system regulation centering on the different functions of the vagus nerve and the importance of cues of safety versus danger; conceptualized by Dr. Stephen Porges.

prefrontal cortex (PFC): The "thinking brain" responsible for executive regulation, abstract reasoning, and voluntary control; loses regulatory control under stress and high threat physiology.

projection: The process of attributing certain thoughts and characteristics to another person when those thoughts and characteristics really represent your interpretation of that person. Most of our opinions are simply our view of ourselves projected onto the world. This phenomenon completely clouds awareness.

psychological reflex: When you're re-exposed to a similar situation that originally created a strong emotional response, your body will automatically respond again in an identical manner.

repetitive unwanted thoughts (RUTs): Intrusive, distressing thoughts ranging from mild to severe. RUTs are universal to all humans, driven by threat states, and exacerbated by suppression, repression, and maladaptive control strategies.

repression: Automatic unconscious suppression. A common response to mental and physical pain, it manifests in untoward behavior.

reprogramming: Learning any skill involves repetition until it becomes permanently embedded in the nervous system. Reprogramming is creating alternate pathways to a stimulus.

safety physiology: The physiological state of relaxation and restoration, dominated by parasympathetic nervous system activity (especially the vagus nerve), lowering stress hormones, and promoting healing, social connection, and neuroplasticity.

sapiocortex: The highest region of the prefrontal cortex responsible for abstract thinking and wisdom, most vulnerable to stress-induced shutdown; term coined by Dr. DR Clawson to describe the areas involved in the highest cognitive functions. Includes dlPFC and several surrounding regions.

schadenfreude: Feeling pleasure or satisfaction in response to another's misfortune. Rooted in survival circuitry, this uncontrollable reaction activates reward pathways such as the ventral striatum, and is addictive because it temporarily reduces one's own pain. Active schadenfreude is deliberate behavior intended to cause pain to others for personal relief or satisfaction, including bullying or "cutting down the tall poppy." See *tall poppy syndrome*.

self-esteem: The subjective sense of personal worth or value, often distinguished from confidence (which is skill-based) and ego (which is defensive). High self-esteem reflects self-acceptance rather than perpetual achievement. It is the antithesis of ego.

sociostasis: A concept developed by Dr. Sue Carter, which she defines as the biologically anchored state of physiological stability maintained by social bonds, central to health, healing, and resilience.

somatosensory component: Pain has both an emotional (affective) and physical component. The part of the nervous system that localizes the physical sensation to the body part is called the somatosensory component.

suppression: Conscious effort to avoid unpleasant thoughts.

sympathetic nervous system (SNS): A branch of the autonomic nervous system that activates the body's "fight-or-flight" response under stress, increasing heart rate, blood pressure, breathing rate, and pupil size while slowing digestion. Its nerves use norepinephrine and epinephrine to rapidly redirect energy to essential functions needed for survival.

tall poppy syndrome (TPS): The drive to resent, diminish, or undermine those perceived as more successful; fueled by envy and often a source of active schadenfreude

threat physiology: A state of heightened stress arousal: increased sympathetic tone, stress hormones, and vulnerability to illness. It often manifests as anxiety, anger, pain, or rapid, repetitive thinking.

trampoline effect: Based on the "ironic effect"—the harder you push down or suppress a thought, the more violently it rebounds, strengthening repetitive unwanted thoughts.

trigger: The nervous system's sustained chemical response to unrelenting thoughts or other sensations, which can also create symptoms based on prior traumas.

vagal tone: A marker of parasympathetic ("rest and digest") function and safety. Higher tone means greater resilience and capacity to recover.

vagus nerve (cranial X): The tenth and longest cranial nerve, and a core part of the parasympathetic nervous system. It connects to every organ in the body. Plays a major role in the regulation of involuntary functions such as blood pressure, heart rate, and digestion.

ventromedial PFC (vmPFC): Bridges rational cognition with emotion by integrating feeling states and supporting flexible emotional regulation in safe states; disrupted by chronic threat.

Recommended Reading

Allen, David. *Getting Things Done: The Art of Stress-Free Productivity.* Penguin, 2015.

Burns, Dr. David D. *Feeling Good: The New Mood Therapy.* William Morrow, 1999.

Coyle, Daniel. *The Talent Code: Greatness Isn't Born. It's Grown. Here's How. Bantam, 2009.*

de Mello, Anthony. *The Way to Love: The Last Meditations of Anthony de Mello.* Image, 1995.

Gordon, Dr. Thomas. *Parent Effectiveness Training: The Proven Program for Raising Responsible Children.* Harmony, 2000.

Lebell, Sharon. *The Art of Living: The Classical Manual on Virtue, Happiness, and Effectiveness.* HarperOne, 2007.

Luskin, Dr. Fred. *Forgive for Good: A Proven Prescription for Health and Happiness.* HarperOne, 2003.

Pennebaker, Dr. James. *Opening Up by Writing It Down: How Expressive Writing Improves Health and Eases Pain* (3rd edition). The Guildford Press, 2016.

Porges, Stephen W. *The Pocket Guide to the Polyvagal Theory: The Transformative Power of Feeling Safe.* W. W. Norton, 2017.

Seigel, Dr. Bernie. *Love, Medicine & Miracles.* HarperPerennial, 1998.

Notes

Introduction

1. Christina Alexandra Löw et al., "Self-Criticism and Psychotherapy Outcome: A Systematic Review and Meta-Analysis," *Clinical Psychology Review* 75 (February 2020): 101808, https://doi.org/10.1016/j.cpr.2019.101808.
2. Amy F. T. Arnsten, "Stress Signaling Pathways That Impair Prefrontal Cortex Structure and Function," *Nature Reviews Neuroscience* 10, no. 6 (2009): 410–22, https://doi.org/10.1038/nrn2648.
3. A. M. Ruscio et al., "The Epidemiology of Obsessive-Compulsive Disorder in the National Comorbidity Survey Replication," *Molecular Psychiatry* 15, no. 1 (2010): 53–63, https://doi.org/10.1038/mp.2008.94.
4. Kate Allsopp et al., "Heterogeneity in Psychiatric Diagnostic Classification," *Psychiatry Research* 279 (September 2019): 15–22, https://doi.org/10.1016/j.psychres.2019.07.005.
5. Isaac R. Galatzer-Levy and Richard A. Bryant, "636,120 Ways to Have Posttraumatic Stress Disorder," *Perspectives on Psychological Science* 8, no. 6 (2013): 651–62, https://doi.org/10.1177/1745691613504115.
6. Charles M. Olbert et al., "Quantifying Heterogeneity Attributable to Polythetic Diagnostic Criteria: Theoretical Framework and Empirical Application," *Journal of Abnormal Psychology* 123, no. 2 (2014): 452–62, https://doi.org/10.1037/a0036068.
7. Rebecca Morrison and Rory C. O'Connor, "A Systematic Review of the Relationship Between Rumination and Suicidality," *Suicide and Life-Threatening Behavior* 38, no. 5 (2008): 523–38, https://doi.org/10.1521/suli.2008.38.5.523.
8. Gary M. Franklin et al., "Outcome of Lumbar Fusion in Washington State Workers' Compensation," *Spine* 19, no. 17 (1994): 1897–903, https://doi.org/10.1097/00007632-199409000-00005.
9. Howard Schubiner and Michael Betzold, *Unlearn Your Pain: A 28-Day Process to Reprogram Your Brain*, 4th edition (Mind Body Publishing, 2022).
10. David Hanscom, *Back in Control: A Surgeon's Roadmap Out of Chronic Pain*, 2nd edition (Vertus Press, 2017).
11. Stephen W. Porges, *The Polyvagal Theory: Neurophysiological Foundations of Emotions, Attachment, Communication, and Self-Regulation*, 1st edition, The Norton Series on Interpersonal Neurobiology (W. W. Norton, 2011).
12. C. Sue Carter, "Oxytocin Pathways and the Evolution of Human Behavior," *Annual Review of Psychology* 65, no. 1 (2014): 17–39, https://doi.org/10.1146/annurev-psych-010213-115110.

Chapter 1: The Curse of Consciousness

1. David Veale et al., "Risk Assessment and Management in Obsessive-Compulsive Disorder," *Advances in Psychiatric Treatment* 15, no. 5 (2009): 332–43, https://doi.org/10.1192/apt.bp.107.004705.
2. Weifeng Zhang et al., "Role of Neuroinflammation in Neurodegeneration Development," *Signal Transduction and Targeted Therapy* 8, no. 1 (2023): 267, https://doi.org/10.1038/s41392-023-01486-5.
3. Naomi I. Eisenberger et al., "Does Rejection Hurt? An fMRI Study of Social Exclusion," *Science* 302, no. 5643 (2003): 290–92, https://doi.org/10.1126/science.1089134.

4. A. R. Mansour et al., "Chronic Pain: The Role of Learning and Brain Plasticity," *Restorative Neurology and Neuroscience* 32, no. 1 (2014): 129–39, https://doi.org/10.3233/RNN-139003.
5. Haeorum Park et al., "Anterior Insular Cortex Glutamate-Glutamine (Glx) Levels Predict General Psychopathology via Heightened Error Sensitivity," *Frontiers in Neuroscience* 19 (July 2025): 1592015, https://doi.org/10.3389/fnins.2025.1592015.
6. Firdaus S. Dhabhar, "The Short-Term Stress Response—Mother Nature's Mechanism for Enhancing Protection and Performance Under Conditions of Threat, Challenge, and Opportunity," *Frontiers in Neuroendocrinology* 49 (April 2018): 175–92, https://doi.org/10.1016/j.yfrne.2018.03.004.
7. Richard D. Lane et al., "Biased Competition Favoring Physical Over Emotional Pain: A Possible Explanation for the Link Between Early Adversity and Chronic Pain," *Psychosomatic Medicine* 80, no. 9 (2018): 880–90, https://doi.org/10.1097/PSY.0000000000000640.
8. Daniel M. Wegner et al., "Paradoxical Effects of Thought Suppression," *Journal of Personality and Social Psychology* 53, no. 1 (1987): 5–13, https://doi.org/10.1037/0022-3514.53.1.5.
9. Laura Smart and Daniel M. Wegner, "Covering Up What Can't Be Seen: Concealable Stigma and Mental Control," *Journal of Personality and Social Psychology* 77, no. 3 (1999): 474–86, https://doi.org/10.1037/0022-3514.77.3.474.
10. Daniel M. Wegner and Thalia Wheatley, "Apparent Mental Causation: Sources of the Experience of Will," *American Psychologist* 54, no. 7 (1999): 480–92, https://doi.org/10.1037/0003-066X.54.7.480.
11. John A. Bargh and Ezequiel Morsella, "The Unconscious Mind," *Perspectives on Psychological Science* 3, no. 1 (2008): 73–79, https://doi.org/10.1111/j.1745-6916.2008.00064.x.
12. Lydia R. Temoshok et al., "Type C Coping, Alexithymia, and Heart Rate Reactivity Are Associated Independently and Differentially with Specific Immune Mechanisms Linked to HIV Progression," *Brain, Behavior, and Immunity* 22, no. 5 (2008): 781–92, https://doi.org/10.1016/j.bbi.2008.02.003.
13. M. Namnyak et al., "'Stockholm Syndrome': Psychiatric Diagnosis or Urban Myth?," *Acta Psychiatrica Scandinavica* 117, no. 1 (2008): 4–11, https://doi.org/10.1111/j.1600-0447.2007.01112.x.
14. Stephen W. Porges, "The Polyvagal Perspective," *Biological Psychology* 74, no. 2 (2007): 116–43, https://doi.org/10.1016/j.biopsycho.2006.06.009.
15. Rebecca Bailey et al., "Appeasement: Replacing Stockholm Syndrome as a Definition of a Survival Strategy," *European Journal of Psychotraumatology* 14, no. 1 (2023): 2161038, https://doi.org/10.1080/20008066.2022.2161038.
16. George M. Slavich and Michael R. Irwin, "From Stress to Inflammation and Major Depressive Disorder: A Social Signal Transduction Theory of Depression," *Psychological Bulletin* 140, no. 3 (2014): 774–815, https://doi.org/10.1037/a0035302.
17. William E. Copeland et al., "Adult Psychiatric Outcomes of Bullying and Being Bullied by Peers in Childhood and Adolescence," *JAMA Psychiatry* 70, no. 4 (2013): 419, https://doi.org/10.1001/jamapsychiatry.2013.504.

Chapter 2: The Physiology of Feeling Unsafe

1. Carl Lange and William James, "The Emotions," Williams & Wilkens Company, 1922, https://ia801604.us.archive.org/4/items/emotions00lang/emotions00lang.pdf.
2. Joseph E. LeDoux, "Emotion Circuits in the Brain," *Annual Review of Neuroscience* 23, no. 1 (2000): 155–84, https://doi.org/10.1146/annurev.neuro.23.1.155.
3. Rolf-Detlef Treede et al., "Chronic Pain as a Symptom or a Disease: The IASP Classification of Chronic Pain for the International Classification of Diseases (ICD-11)," *Pain* 160, no. 1 (2019): 19–27, https://doi.org/10.1097/j.pain.0000000000001384.
4. A. R. Mansour et al., "Chronic Pain: The Role of Learning and Brain Plasticity," *Restorative Neurology and Neuroscience* 32, no. 1 (2014): 129–39, https://doi.org/10.3233/RNN-139003.

5. Robert K. Naviaux, "Metabolic Features of the Cell Danger Response," *Mitochondrion* 16 (May 2014): 7–17, https://doi.org/10.1016/j.mito.2013.08.006.
6. Robert K. Naviaux et al., "Low-Dose Suramin in Autism Spectrum Disorder: A Small, Phase I/II, Randomized Clinical Trial," *Annals of Clinical and Translational Neurology* 4, no. 7 (2017): 491–505, https://doi.org/10.1002/acn3.424.
7. Ernest Becker, *The Denial of Death* (Free Press, 1997).
8. Paul W. Brand and Philip Yancey, *Pain: The Gift Nobody Wants*, 1st edition (HarperCollins Publishers; Zondervan, 1993).
9. Ashkahn Golshani et al., "Congenital Indifference to Pain: An Illustrated Case Report and Literature Review," *Journal of Radiology Case Reports* 8, no. 8 (2014): 16–23, https://doi.org/10.3941/jrcr.v8i8.2194.
10. Patrick H. Finan et al., "The Association of Sleep and Pain: An Update and a Path Forward," *Journal of Pain* 14, no. 12 (2013): 1539–52, https://doi.org/10.1016/j.jpain.2013.08.007.
11. Maayan Agmon and Galit Armon, "Increased Insomnia Symptoms Predict the Onset of Back Pain Among Employed Adults," *PLoS ONE* 9, no. 8 (2014): e103591, https://doi.org/10.1371/journal.pone.0103591.
12. Y. Fan et al., "The Narcissistic Self and Its Psychological and Neural Correlates: An Exploratory fMRI Study," *Psychological Medicine* 41, no. 8 (2011): 1641–50, https://doi.org/10.1017/S003329171000228X.
13. Samuel J. DeWitt et al., "The Hyper-Sentient Addict: An Exteroception Model of Addiction," *American Journal of Drug and Alcohol Abuse* 41, no. 5 (2015): 374–81, https://doi.org/10.3109/00952990.2015.1049701.
14. A. D. Craig, "How Do You Feel? Interoception: The Sense of the Physiological Condition of the Body," *Nature Reviews Neuroscience* 3, no. 8 (2002): 655–66, https://doi.org/10.1038/nrn894.
15. Stephen W. Porges, personal communication (October 21, 2025).
16. Stephen W. Porges, "The Polyvagal Perspective," *Biological Psychology* 74, no. 2 (2007): 116–43, https://doi.org/10.1016/j.biopsycho.2006.06.009.
17. Stephen W. Porges, "The Polyvagal Theory: Phylogenetic Substrates of a Social Nervous System," *International Journal of Psychophysiology* 42, no. 2 (2001): 123–46, https://doi.org/10.1016/S0167-8760(01)00162-3.
18. Frederico A. C. Azevedo et al., "Equal Numbers of Neuronal and Nonneuronal Cells Make the Human Brain an Isometrically Scaled-Up Primate Brain," *Journal of Comparative Neurology* 513, no. 5 (2009): 532–41, https://doi.org/10.1002/cne.21974.
19. G. Lorimer Moseley and David S. Butler, "Fifteen Years of Explaining Pain: The Past, Present, and Future," *Journal of Pain* 16, no. 9 (2015): 807–13, https://doi.org/10.1016/j.jpain.2015.05.005.
20. Julian F. Thayer et al., "The Relationship of Autonomic Imbalance, Heart Rate Variability and Cardiovascular Disease Risk Factors," *International Journal of Cardiology* 141, no. 2 (2010): 122–31, https://doi.org/10.1016/j.ijcard.2009.09.543.
21. Christian Lopez Blanco and William J. Tyler, "The Vagus Nerve: A Cornerstone for Mental Health and Performance Optimization in Recreation and Elite Sports," *Frontiers in Psychology* 16 (July 2025): 1639866, https://doi.org/10.3389/fpsyg.2025.1639866.
22. Stephen Porges, "Neuroception: A Subconscious System for Detecting Threats and Safety. Zero to Three," unpublished manuscript, Zero to Three, 2004.
23. Robert Dantzer et al., "Resilience and Immunity," *Brain, Behavior, and Immunity* 74 (November 2018): 28–42, https://doi.org/10.1016/j.bbi.2018.08.010.
24. C. Sue Carter, "Oxytocin Pathways and the Evolution of Human Behavior," *Annual Review of Psychology* 65, no. 1 (2014): 17–39, https://doi.org/10.1146/annurev-psych-010213-115110.
25. Markus Heinrichs et al., "Oxytocin, Vasopressin, and Human Social Behavior," *Frontiers in Neuroendocrinology* 30, no. 4 (2009): 548–57, https://doi.org/10.1016/j.yfrne.2009.05.005.

26. Steven W. Cole, "The Conserved Transcriptional Response to Adversity," *Current Opinion in Behavioral Sciences* 28 (August 2019): 31–37, https://doi.org/10.1016/j.cobeha.2019.01.008.
27. Douglas Nemecek, *Cigna U.S. Loneliness Report* (Cigna Insurance, 2018), 61.
28. Chen Lyu et al., "Social Isolation Changes and Long-Term Outcomes Among Older Adults," *JAMA Network Open* 7, no. 7 (2024): e2424519, https://doi.org/10.1001/jamanetworkopen.2024.24519.

Chapter 3: The Survival Quartet: Anxiety, Envy, Anger, Schadenfreude

1. Hidehiko Takahashi et al., "When Your Gain Is My Pain and Your Pain Is My Gain: Neural Correlates of Envy and Schadenfreude," *Science* 323, no. 5916 (2009): 937–39, https://doi.org/10.1126/science.1165604.
2. Eric L. Garland et al., "Thought Suppression as a Mediator of the Association Between Depressed Mood and Prescription Opioid Craving Among Chronic Pain Patients," *Journal of Behavioral Medicine* 39, no. 1 (2016): 128–38, https://doi.org/10.1007/s10865-015-9675-9.
3. Amy F. T. Arnsten, "Stress Signalling Pathways That Impair Prefrontal Cortex Structure and Function," *Nature Reviews Neuroscience* 10, no. 6 (2009): 410–22, https://doi.org/10.1038/nrn2648.
4. Donald O. Hebb, *The Organization of Behavior: A Neuropsychological Theory*, 11. [print.] (Wiley, 1974).
5. Suzana Herculano-Houzel, "Scaling of Brain Metabolism with a Fixed Energy Budget per Neuron: Implications for Neuronal Activity, Plasticity and Evolution," *PLoS ONE* 6, no. 3 (2011): e17514, https://doi.org/10.1371/journal.pone.0017514.
6. Amy F. T. Arnsten, "Stress Signalling Pathways That Impair Prefrontal Cortex Structure and Function," *Nature Reviews Neuroscience* 10, no. 6 (2009): 410–22, https://doi.org/10.1038/nrn2648.
7. Amy F. T. Arnsten, "Stress Signalling Pathways That Impair Prefrontal Cortex Structure and Function," *Nature Reviews Neuroscience* 10, no. 6 (2009): 410–22, https://doi.org/10.1038/nrn2648.
8. Vinod Menon and Lucina Q. Uddin, "Saliency, Switching, Attention and Control: A Network Model of Insula Function," *Brain Structure and Function* 214, nos. 5–6 (2010): 655–67, https://doi.org/10.1007/s00429-010-0262-0.
9. Hidehiko Takahashi et al., "When Your Gain Is My Pain and Your Pain Is My Gain: Neural Correlates of Envy and Schadenfreude," *Science* 323, no. 5916 (2009): 937–39, https://doi.org/10.1126/science.1165604.
10. Birgit A. Völlm et al., "Neuronal Correlates of Theory of Mind and Empathy: A Functional Magnetic Resonance Imaging Study in a Nonverbal Task," *NeuroImage* 29, no. 1 (2006): 90–98, https://doi.org/10.1016/j.neuroimage.2005.07.022.
11. David S. Chester and C. Nathan DeWall, "Personality Correlates of Revenge-Seeking: Multidimensional Links to Physical Aggression, Impulsivity, and Aggressive Pleasure," *Aggressive Behavior* 44, no. 3 (2018): 235–45, https://doi.org/10.1002/ab.21746.
12. Mina Cikara et al., "Us and Them: Intergroup Failures of Empathy," *Current Directions in Psychological Science* 20, no. 3 (2011): 149–53, https://doi.org/10.1177/0963721411408713.
13. Jeremy Hogeveen et al., "Power Changes How the Brain Responds to Others," *Journal of Experimental Psychology: General* 143, no. 2 (2014): 755–62, https://doi.org/10.1037/a0033477.
14. N. T. Feather, "Attitudes Towards the High Achiever: The Fall of the Tall Poppy," *Australian Journal of Psychology* 41, no. 3 (1989): 239–67, https://doi.org/10.1080/00049538908260088.
15. Douglas Garland and Brian Schwartz, *The Tall Poppy Syndrome: The Joy of Cutting Others Down*, Rev. 1.13, ed. Irene Chambers (2022).
16. Livy et al., *The Early History of Rome: Books I–V of the History of Rome from Its Foundations*, Penguin Classics (Penguin Books, 2002).
17. Ryu Takizawa et al., "Adult Health Outcomes of Childhood Bullying Victimization: Evidence from a Five-Decade Longitudinal British Birth Cohort," *American Journal of Psychiatry* 171, no. 7 (2014): 777–84, https://doi.org/10.1176/appi.ajp.2014.13101401.

18. R. Takizawa et al., "Bullying Victimization in Childhood Predicts Inflammation and Obesity at Mid-Life: A Five-Decade Birth Cohort Study," *Psychological Medicine* 45, no. 13 (2015): 2705–15, https://doi.org/10.1017/S0033291715000653.
19. William E. Copeland et al., "Adult Psychiatric Outcomes of Bullying and Being Bullied by Peers in Childhood and Adolescence," *JAMA Psychiatry* 70, no. 4 (2013): 419, https://doi.org/10.1001/jamapsychiatry.2013.504.
20. Melanie Neumann et al., "Empathy Decline and Its Reasons: A Systematic Review of Studies with Medical Students and Residents," *Academic Medicine* 86, no. 8 (2011): 996–1009, https://doi.org/10.1097/ACM.0b013e318221e615.
21. Henrietta Bolló et al., "The Role of Subjective and Objective Social Status in the Generation of Envy," *Frontiers in Psychology* 11 (December 2020): 513495, https://doi.org/10.3389/fpsyg.2020.513495.
22. Douglas Garland and Brian Schwartz, *The Tall Poppy Syndrome: The Joy of Cutting Others Down*, Rev. 1.13, ed. Irene Chambers (2022).
23. Susan Nolen-Hoeksema et al., "Rethinking Rumination," *Perspectives on Psychological Science* 3, no. 5 (2008): 400–24, https://doi.org/10.1111/j.1745-6924.2008.00088.x.
24. Shigeru Miyagawa et al., "Linguistic Capacity Was Present in the *Homo Sapiens* Population 135 Thousand Years Ago," *Frontiers in Psychology* 16 (March 2025): 1503900, https://doi.org/10.3389/fpsyg.2025.1503900.

Chapter 4: Brainwashed by Our Lives

1. B. Draganski et al., "Temporal and Spatial Dynamics of Brain Structure Changes During Extensive Learning," *Journal of Neuroscience* 26, no. 23 (2006): 6314–17, https://doi.org/10.1523/JNEUROSCI.4628-05.2006.
2. B. Draganski et al., "Temporal and Spatial Dynamics of Brain Structure Changes During Extensive Learning," *Journal of Neuroscience* 26, no. 23 (2006): 6314–17, https://doi.org/10.1523/JNEUROSCI.4628-05.2006.
3. David A. Seminowicz et al., "Effective Treatment of Chronic Low Back Pain in Humans Reverses Abnormal Brain Anatomy and Function," *Journal of Neuroscience* 31, no. 20 (2011): 7540–50, https://doi.org/10.1523/JNEUROSCI.5280-10.2011.
4. Daniel Coyle, *The Talent Code: Greatness Isn't Born. It's Grown. Here's How* (Bantam Books, 2009).
5. Robert A. Boakes, *Pavlov's Legacy: How and What Animals Learn*, 1st edition (Cambridge University Press, 2023), https://doi.org/10.1017/9781009057530.
6. David Eagleman, *Livewired: The Inside Story of the Ever-Changing Brain*, first Vintage Books edition (Vintage Books, 2021).
7. Vincent J. Felitti, "Childhood Sexual Abuse, Depression, and Family Dysfunction in Adult Obese Patients: A Case Control Study," *Southern Medical Journal* 86, no. 7 (1993): 732–36, https://doi.org/10.1097/00007611-199307000-00002.
8. Vincent J Felitti et al., "Relationship of Childhood Abuse and Household Dysfunction to Many of the Leading Causes of Death in Adults," *American Journal of Preventive Medicine* 14, no. 4 (1998): 245–58, https://doi.org/10.1016/S0749-3797(98)00017-8.
9. Jing Shen et al., "The Relationship Between Parental Adverse Childhood Experiences and Offspring Preschool Readiness: The Mediating Role of Psychological Resilience," *BMC Psychology* 13, no. 1 (2025): 136, https://doi.org/10.1186/s40359-025-02408-6.
10. Elizabeth A. Swedo et al., "Adverse Childhood Experiences and Health Conditions and Risk Behaviors Among High School Students—Youth Risk Behavior Survey, United States, 2023," *MMWR Supplements* 73, no. 4 (2024): 39–50, https://doi.org/10.15585/mmwr.su7304a5.

11. Shawn Ratcliff et al., "Adverse Childhood Experiences: Increased Likelihood of Socioeconomic Disadvantages for Young Adults: Article Examines Socioeconomic Disadvantages for Young Adults Who Had Experienced Adverse Childhood Experiences," *Health Affairs* 44, no. 1 (2025): 108–16, https://doi.org/10.1377/hlthaff.2024.00827.
12. Susan Nolen-Hoeksema et al., "Rethinking Rumination," *Perspectives on Psychological Science* 3, no. 5 (2008): 400–424, https://doi.org/10.1111/j.1745-6924.2008.00088.x.
13. Sara King et al., "The Epidemiology of Chronic Pain in Children and Adolescents Revisited: A Systematic Review," *Pain* 152, no. 12 (2011): 2729–38, https://doi.org/10.1016/j.pain.2011.07.016.
14. Gemma García-Soriano et al., "Obsessional Intrusive Thoughts in Children: An Interview Based Study," *Psychology and Psychotherapy: Theory, Research and Practice* 96, no. 1 (2023): 249–62, https://doi.org/10.1111/papt.12437.
15. Freya Mills et al., "A Mixed Studies Systematic Review on the Health and Wellbeing Effects, and Underlying Mechanisms, of Online Support Groups for Chronic Conditions," *Communications Psychology* 3, no. 1 (2025): 40, https://doi.org/10.1038/s44271-025-00217-6.
16. Robert Ferrari and Anthony Science Russell, "Effect of a Symptom Diary on Symptom Frequency and Intensity in Healthy Subjects," *Journal of Rheumatology* 37, no. 11 (2010): 2387–89, https://doi.org/10.3899/jrheum.100513.

Chapter 5: The Illusion of Control

1. Julian B. Rotter, "Generalized Expectancies for Internal Versus External Control of Reinforcement," *Psychological Monographs: General and Applied* 80, no. 1 (1966): 1–28, https://doi.org/10.1037/h0092976.
2. Robert Dantzer et al., "Resilience and Immunity," *Brain, Behavior, and Immunity* 74 (November 2018): 28–42, https://doi.org/10.1016/j.bbi.2018.08.010.
3. Richard M. Ryan and Edward L. Deci, "Self-Determination Theory and the Facilitation of Intrinsic Motivation, Social Development, and Well-Being," *American Psychologist* 55, no. 1 (2000): 68–78, https://doi.org/10.1037/0003-066X.55.1.68.
4. Martin Picard et al., "Mitochondrial Psychobiology: Foundations and Applications," *Current Opinion in Behavioral Sciences* 28 (August 2019): 142–51, https://doi.org/10.1016/j.cobeha.2019.04.015.
5. Steven C. Hayes, *Get Out of Your Mind and into Your Life: The New Acceptance and Commitment Therapy*, 20th anniversary edition (New Harbinger Publications, 2025).
6. Elizabeth T. Gershoff and Andrew Grogan-Kaylor, "Spanking and Child Outcomes: Old Controversies and New Meta-Analyses," *Journal of Family Psychology* 30, no. 4 (2016): 453–69, https://doi.org/10.1037/fam0000191.
7. Harsh Wadhwa et al., "Imposter Syndrome Among Orthopaedic Surgery Residents Is Extremely Common and Disproportionately Affects Female Residents," *JBJS Open Access* 10, no. 2 (2025), https://doi.org/10.2106/JBJS.OA.24.00132.
8. Tore Charles Stiles and Danielle Wright, "Cognitive-Behavioural Treatment of Chronic Pain Conditions," *Nordic Journal of Psychiatry* 62, no. sup47 (2008): 30–36, https://doi.org/10.1080/08039480802315665.
9. Marc L. Berk and Alan C. Monheit, "The Concentration of Health Care Expenditures, Revisited," *Health Affairs* 20, no. 2 (2001): 9–18, https://doi.org/10.1377/hlthaff.20.2.9.
10. Washington State Health Care Authority, Washington State Health Care Cost Transparency Board, Annual Report, Second Substitute House Bill 2457; Section 7(2); Chapter 340; Laws of 2020; Substitute Senate Bill 5589; Section 1(3); Chapter 155; Laws of 2022; Second Engrossed Substitute House Bill 1508; Section 3(1); Chapter 80; Laws of 2024. December 1, 2024 (2024), https://www.hca.wa.gov/assets/program/cost-board-2024-leg-report.pdf.

11. Todd B. Kashdan and Jonathan Rottenberg, "Psychological Flexibility as a Fundamental Aspect of Health," *Clinical Psychology Review* 30, no. 7 (2010): 865–78, https://doi.org/10.1016/j.cpr.2010.03.001.
12. John Pearn, "Hammurabi's Code: A Primary Datum in the Conjoined Professions of Medicine and Law," *Medico-Legal Journal* 84, no. 3 (2016): 125–31, https://doi.org/10.1177/0025817216646038.
13. Patricia Evans, *The Verbally Abusive Relationship: How to Recognize It and How to Respond*, expanded 3rd edition (Adams Media Corporation, 2010).
14. Sarah Miller, "Today's Parents: 'Exhausted, Burned Out and Perpetually Behind,'" *New York Times*, September 14, 2024.
15. Rebecca Morrison and Rory C. O'Connor, "A Systematic Review of the Relationship Between Rumination and Suicidality," *Suicide and Life-Threatening Behavior* 38, no. 5 (2008): 523–38, https://doi.org/10.1521/suli.2008.38.5.523.

Chapter 7: Separate from Your Thoughts

1. Steven C. Hayes et al., "Acceptance and Commitment Therapy: Model, Processes and Outcomes," *Behaviour Research and Therapy* 44, no. 1 (2006): 1–25, https://doi.org/10.1016/j.brat.2005.06.006.
2. Andrea N. Niles et al., "Randomized Controlled Trial of Expressive Writing for Psychological and Physical Health: The Moderating Role of Emotional Expressivity," *Anxiety, Stress, & Coping* 27, no. 1 (2014): 1–17, https://doi.org/10.1080/10615806.2013.802308.
3. Michael C. Anderson et al., "Brain Mechanisms Underlying the Inhibitory Control of Thought," *Nature Reviews Neuroscience* 26, no. 7 (2025): 415–37, https://doi.org/10.1038/s41583-025-00929-y.
4. James W. Pennebaker and Sandra K. Beall, "Confronting a Traumatic Event: Toward an Understanding of Inhibition and Disease," *Journal of Abnormal Psychology* 95, no. 3 (1986): 274–81, https://doi.org/10.1037/0021-843X.95.3.274.
5. Cristina Ottaviani et al., "Physiological Concomitants of Perseverative Cognition: A Systematic Review and Meta-Analysis," *Psychological Bulletin* 142, no. 3 (2016): 231–59, https://doi.org/10.1037/bul0000036.
6. Justin B. Echouffo-Tcheugui et al., "Circulating Cortisol and Cognitive and Structural Brain Measures: The Framingham Heart Study," *Neurology* 91, no. 21 (2018), https://doi.org/10.1212/WNL.0000000000006549.
7. Cristina Ottaviani et al., "Physiological Concomitants of Perseverative Cognition: A Systematic Review and Meta-Analysis," *Psychological Bulletin* 142, no. 3 (2016): 231–59, https://doi.org/10.1037/bul0000036.
8. James A. K. Erskine, "Resistance Can Be Futile: Investigating Behavioural Rebound," *Appetite* 50, nos. 2–3 (2008): 415–21, https://doi.org/10.1016/j.appet.2007.09.006.
9. James W. Pennebaker and Sandra K. Beall, "Confronting a Traumatic Event: Toward an Understanding of Inhibition and Disease," *Journal of Abnormal Psychology* 95, no. 3 (1986): 274–81, https://doi.org/10.1037/0021-843X.95.3.274.
10. James W. Pennebaker and Joshua M. Smyth, *Opening Up by Writing It Down: How Expressive Writing Improves Health and Eases Emotional Pain*, 3rd edition (Guilford Press, 2016).
11. Daniel Wegner, "The Seed of Our Undoing," *Psychological Science Agenda* (American Psychological Association), February 1999.
12. David D. Burns, *Feeling Good: The New Mood Therapy*, 1st edition (HarperCollins Publishers, 1999).
13. Jason S. Moser et al., "Third-Person Self-Talk Facilitates Emotion Regulation Without Engaging Cognitive Control: Converging Evidence from ERP and fMRI," *Scientific Reports* 7, no. 1 (2017): 4519, https://doi.org/10.1038/s41598-017-04047-3.
14. B. Alan Wallace and Tsong-kha-pa Blo-bzang-grags-pa, *The Bridge of Quiescence: Experiencing Tibetan Buddhist Meditation* (Open Court, 1998).

Chapter 8: Calm Your Physiology

1. David D. Burns, *Feeling Good: The New Mood Therapy*, 1st edition (HarperCollins Publishers, 1999).
2. James W. Carson et al., "Forgiveness and Chronic Low Back Pain: A Preliminary Study Examining the Relationship of Forgiveness to Pain, Anger, and Psychological Distress," *Journal of Pain* 6, no. 2 (2005): 84–91, https://doi.org/10.1016/j.jpain.2004.10.012.
3. John E. Sarno, *Healing Back Pain: The Mind-Body Connection*, first Grand Central Publishing trade paperback edition (Grand Central Publishing, 2019).
4. Cavan V. Bonner et al., "Growth Following Adversity Is Rare: Evidence from a Multi-Informant Longitudinal Study of Children and Adolescents," *Journal of Research in Personality* 117 (August 2025): 104628, https://doi.org/10.1016/j.jrp.2025.104628.
5. Shinichi Kumagai et al., "Vagus Nerve Stimulation as a Predictive Coding Modulator That Enhances Feedforward over Feedback Transmission," *Frontiers in Neural Circuits* 19 (April 2025): 1568655, https://doi.org/10.3389/fncir.2025.1568655.
6. Shinichi Kumagai et al., "Vagus Nerve Stimulation as a Predictive Coding Modulator That Enhances Feedforward over Feedback Transmission," *Frontiers in Neural Circuits* 19 (April 2025): 1568655, https://doi.org/10.3389/fncir.2025.1568655.
7. J. Douglas Bremner et al., "Transcutaneous Vagal Nerve Stimulation Blocks Stress-Induced Activation of Interleukin-6 and Interferon-γ in Posttraumatic Stress Disorder: A Double-Blind, Randomized, Sham-Controlled Trial," *Brain, Behavior, & Immunity—Health* 9 (December 2020): 100138, https://doi.org/10.1016/j.bbih.2020.100138.
8. Stephen Porges, "Unyte," SSP Resources, SSP Protocol, n.d., https://integratedlistening.com/polyvagal-theory/porges/.
9. Hsiangkuo Yuan and Stephen D. Silberstein, "Vagus Nerve and Vagus Nerve Stimulation, a Comprehensive Review: Part II," *Headache: The Journal of Head and Face Pain* 56, no. 2 (2016): 259–66, https://doi.org/10.1111/head.12650.
10. Maayan Agmon and Galit Armon, "Increased Insomnia Symptoms Predict the Onset of Back Pain Among Employed Adults," *PLoS ONE* 9, no. 8 (2014): e103591, https://doi.org/10.1371/journal.pone.0103591.
11. Patrick H. Finan et al., "The Association of Sleep and Pain: An Update and a Path Forward," *Journal of Pain* 14, no. 12 (2013): 1539–52, https://doi.org/10.1016/j.jpain.2013.08.007.
12. Marcus O. Harrington et al., "Losing Control: Sleep Deprivation Impairs the Suppression of Unwanted Thoughts," *Clinical Psychological Science* 9, no. 1 (2021): 97–113, https://doi.org/10.1177/2167702620951511.
13. Jung A. Eom et al., "Diet-Regulating Microbiota and Host Immune System in Liver Disease," *International Journal of Molecular Sciences* 22, no. 12 (2021): 6326, https://doi.org/10.3390/ijms22126326.
14. Valter D. Longo and Satchidananda Panda, "Fasting, Circadian Rhythms, and Time-Restricted Feeding in Healthy Lifespan," *Cell Metabolism* 23, no. 6 (2016): 1048–59, https://doi.org/10.1016/j.cmet.2016.06.001.
15. Robert H. Lustig, ed., *Fat Chance: Beating the Odds Against Sugar, Processed Food, Obesity, and Disease*, A Plume Book (Plume, 2014).
16. Alona Pulde et al., *The Forks Over Knives Plan: How to Transition to the Lifesaving, Whole-Food, Plant-Based Diet* (Atria Books, 2018).
17. Carlos Augusto Monteiro et al., "The UN Decade of Nutrition, the NOVA Food Classification and the Trouble with Ultra-Processing," *Public Health Nutrition* 21, no. 1 (2018): 5–17, https://doi.org/10.1017/S1368980017000234.
18. Thibault Fiolet et al., "Consumption of Ultra-Processed Foods and Cancer Risk: Results from NutriNet-Santé Prospective Cohort," *BMJ*, February 14, 2018, k322, https://doi.org/10.1136/bmj.k322.

19. Fiona C. Bull et al., "World Health Organization 2020 Guidelines on Physical Activity and Sedentary Behaviour," *British Journal of Sports Medicine* 54, no. 24 (2020): 1451–62, https://doi.org/10.1136/bjsports-2020-102955.
20. U.S. Department of Health and Human Services, "Physical Activity Guidelines for Americans," 2nd edition, Washington, DC: U.S. Department of Health and Human Services, 2018, https://odphp.health.gov/sites/default/files/2019-09/Physical_Activity_Guidelines_2nd_edition.pdf.
21. Ulf Ekelund et al., "Dose-Response Associations Between Accelerometry Measured Physical Activity and Sedentary Time and All-Cause Mortality: Systematic Review and Harmonized Meta-Analysis," *BMJ*, (August 21, 2019), l4570, https://doi.org/10.1136/bmj.l4570.
22. Frank W. Booth et al., "Lack of Exercise Is a Major Cause of Chronic Diseases," *Comprehensive Physiology* 2, no. 2 (2012): 1143–211, https://doi.org/10.1002/j.2040-4603.2012.tb00425.x.
23. George Mammen and Guy Faulkner, "Physical Activity and the Prevention of Depression," *American Journal of Preventive Medicine* 45, no. 5 (2013): 649–57, https://doi.org/10.1016/j.amepre.2013.08.001.
24. Felipe B. Schuch et al., "Exercise as a Treatment for Depression: A Meta-Analysis Adjusting for Publication Bias," *Journal of Psychiatric Research* 77 (June 2016): 42–51, https://doi.org/10.1016/j.jpsychires.2016.02.023.
25. Bente K. Pedersen and Mark A. Febbraio, "Muscles, Exercise and Obesity: Skeletal Muscle as a Secretory Organ," *Nature Reviews Endocrinology* 8, no. 8 (2012): 457–65, https://doi.org/10.1038/nrendo.2012.49.
26. Alfonso J. Cruz-Jentoft et al., "Sarcopenia: Revised European Consensus on Definition and Diagnosis," *Age and Ageing* 48, no. 1 (2019): 16–31, https://doi.org/10.1093/ageing/afy169.
27. Ming-Dao Deng, *365 Tao: Daily Meditations*, 1st edition (HarperCollins Publishers, 1992).
28. Rita Z. Goldstein and Nora D. Volkow, "Dysfunction of the Prefrontal Cortex in Addiction: Neuroimaging Findings and Clinical Implications," *Nature Reviews Neuroscience* 12, no. 11 (2011): 652–69, https://doi.org/10.1038/nrn3119.
29. Alexander Neumeister et al., "Neural and Behavioral Responses to Tryptophan Depletion in Unmedicated Patients with Remitted Major Depressive Disorder and Controls," *Archives of General Psychiatry* 61, no. 8 (2004): 765, https://doi.org/10.1001/archpsyc.61.8.765.
30. David D. Burns, *Ten Days to Self-Esteem* (Quill, 1993).
31. Tait D. Shanafelt et al., "Changes in Burnout and Satisfaction with Work-Life Integration in Physicians During the First 2 Years of the COVID-19 Pandemic," *Mayo Clinic Proceedings* 97, no. 12 (2022): 2248–58, https://doi.org/10.1016/j.mayocp.2022.09.002.

Chapter 9: Soften Your Ego

1. Kayo Takahashi et al., "Imaging the Passionate Stage of Romantic Love by Dopamine Dynamics," *Frontiers in Human Neuroscience* 9 (April 2015), https://doi.org/10.3389/fnhum.2015.00191.
2. Fran Lebowitz, "Goodreads," Quotable Quotes, n.d., https://www.goodreads.com/quotes/147637-romantic-love-is-mental-illness-but-it-s-a-pleasurable-one.
3. Cavan V. Bonner et al., "Growth Following Adversity Is Rare: Evidence from a Multi-Informant Longitudinal Study of Children and Adolescents," *Journal of Research in Personality* 117 (August 2025): 104628, https://doi.org/10.1016/j.jrp.2025.104628.
4. Paul C. Gorski, "Racial Battle Fatigue and Activist Burnout in Racial Justice Activists of Color at Predominately White Colleges and Universities," *Race Ethnicity and Education* 22, no. 1 (2019): 1–20, https://doi.org/10.1080/13613324.2018.1497966.
5. Joseph Campbell et al., *The Power of Myth* (Anchor Books Doubleday, 1991).

6. Lydia Morris and Warren Mansell, "A Systematic Review of the Relationship Between Rigidity/Flexibility and Transdiagnostic Cognitive and Behavioral Processes That Maintain Psychopathology," *Journal of Experimental Psychopathology* 9, no. 3 (2018): 2043808718779431, https://doi.org/10.1177/2043808718779431.
7. David D. Burns, *Feeling Good: The New Mood Therapy*, 1st edition (HarperCollins Publishers, 1999).
8. David D. Burns, *Feeling Good: The New Mood Therapy*, 1st edition (HarperCollins Publishers, 1999).
9. Sharon Lebell, *The Art of Living: The Classical Manual on Virtue, Happiness, and Effectiveness* (HarperCollins Publishers, 2007).
10. Anthony de Mello, *The Way to Love: The Last Meditations of Anthony de Mello* (Doubleday, 1995).
11. Joseph Telushkin, *Words That Hurt, Words That Heal: How to Choose Words Wisely and Well* (Harper, 2000).

Chapter 10: Rebuild Your Brain

1. Timothy D. Wilson and Elizabeth W. Dunn, "Self-Knowledge: Its Limits, Value, and Potential for Improvement," *Annual Review of Psychology* 55, no. 1 (2004): 493–518, https://doi.org/10.1146/annurev.psych.55.090902.141954.
2. R. A. I. Bethlehem et al., "Brain Charts for the Human Lifespan," *Nature* 604, no. 7906 (2022): 525–33, https://doi.org/10.1038/s41586-022-04554-y.
3. A. D. (Bud) Craig, "How Do You Feel—Now? The Anterior Insula and Human Awareness," *Nature Reviews Neuroscience* 10, no. 1 (2009): 59–70, https://doi.org/10.1038/nrn2555.
4. Robert K. Naviaux, "Metabolic Features of the Cell Danger Response," *Mitochondrion* 16 (May 2014): 7–17, https://doi.org/10.1016/j.mito.2013.08.006.
5. Andrea Irazoki et al., "Disruption of Mitochondrial Dynamics Triggers Muscle Inflammation Through Interorganellar Contacts and Mitochondrial DNA Mislocation," *Nature Communications* 14, no. 1 (2023): 108, https://doi.org/10.1038/s41467-022-35732-1.
6. Emily M. Zitek and Alexander H. Jordan, "Psychological Entitlement Predicts Failure to Follow Instructions," *Social Psychological and Personality Science* 10, no. 2 (2019): 172–80, https://doi.org/10.1177/1948550617729885.
7. Yilu Wang et al., "Altruistic Behaviors Relieve Physical Pain," *Proceedings of the National Academy of Sciences* 117, no. 2 (2020): 950–58, https://doi.org/10.1073/pnas.1911861117.
8. Jaak Panksepp, "Neuroevolutionary Sources of Laughter and Social Joy: Modeling Primal Human Laughter in Laboratory Rats," *Behavioural Brain Research* 182, no. 2 (2007): 231–44, https://doi.org/10.1016/j.bbr.2007.02.015.
9. Clair Cain Miller, "Today's Parents: 'Exhausted, Burned Out and Perpetually Behind,'" The Upshot, *New York Times*, September 14, 2024, https://www.nytimes.com/2024/09/14/upshot/parents-stress-murthy-warning.html?unlocked_article_code=1.1U8.nW65.f0KtponEeVuO&smid=url-share.
10. Marco Iacoboni, "Imitation, Empathy, and Mirror Neurons," *Annual Review of Psychology* 60, no. 1 (2009): 653–70, https://doi.org/10.1146/annurev.psych.60.110707.163604.
11. David Allen, *Getting Things Done: The Art of Stress-Free Productivity*, revised edition, with James M. Fallows (Penguin Books, 2015).
12. D. W. Dunstan et al., "Television Viewing Time and Mortality: The Australian Diabetes, Obesity and Lifestyle Study (AusDiab)," *Circulation* 121, no. 3 (2010): 384–91, https://doi.org/10.1161/CIRCULATIONAHA.109.894824.
13. "World Health Organization Commission on Social Connection. 2025. *Report of the WHO Commission on Social Connection*. Geneva: World Health Organization," 2025.
14. Robert J. Waldinger and Marc S. Schulz, *The Good Life: Lessons from the World's Longest Scientific Study of Happiness*, first Simon & Schuster hardcover edition (Simon & Schuster, 2023).

15. Steven W. Cole, "Human Social Genomics," *PLoS Genetics* 10, no. 8 (2014): e1004601, https://doi.org/10.1371/journal.pgen.1004601.
16. C. Sue Carter and Stephen W. Porges, "The Biochemistry of Love: An Oxytocin Hypothesis: Science & Society Series on Sex and Science," *EMBO Reports* 14, no. 1 (2013): 12–16, https://doi.org/10.1038/embor.2012.191.
17. John W. Burns et al., "Temporal Associations Between Spouse Criticism/Hostility and Pain Among Patients with Chronic Pain: A Within-Couple Daily Diary Study," *Pain* 154, no. 12 (2013): 2715–21, https://doi.org/10.1016/j.pain.2013.07.053.
18. Peter Schnohr et al., "Various Leisure-Time Physical Activities Associated with Widely Divergent Life Expectancies: The Copenhagen City Heart Study," *Mayo Clinic Proceedings* 93, no. 12 (2018): 1775–85, https://doi.org/10.1016/j.mayocp.2018.06.025.
19. Yue Xu et al., "Association Between Tennis Training Experience and Executive Function in Children Aged 8–12," *Frontiers in Human Neuroscience* 16 (August 2022): 924809, https://doi.org/10.3389/fnhum.2022.924809.

Chapter 11: Awareness Is All You Need

1. Anthony de Mello, *The Way to Love: The Last Meditations of Anthony de Mello* (Doubleday, 1995).
2. Hugh King, *Motorcycle Mania 3: Jesse James Rides Again*, n.d., https://www.imdb.com/title/tt0382858/.
3. Daniel J. Levitin, *I Heard There Was a Secret Chord: Music as Medicine* (W. W. Norton & Company, 2025).
4. Ergos Institute, "Somatic Experiencing," n.d., https://www.somaticexperiencing.com/somatic-experiencing.
5. Paul Gilbert, *The Compassionate Mind: A New Approach to Life's Challenges* (Constable, 2010).
6. Russell L. Kolts, ed., *Experiencing Compassion-Focused Therapy from the Inside Out: A Self-Practice/Self-Reflection Workbook for Therapists* (Guilford Press, 2018).
7. Bstan-'dzin-rgya-mtsho and Howard C. Cutler, *The Art of Happiness: A Handbook for Living*, first Riverhead trade paperback edition (Riverhead Books, 2020).
8. Fabio Giommi et al., "The (In)Flexible Self: Psychopathology, Mindfulness, and Neuroscience," *International Journal of Clinical and Health Psychology* 23, no. 4 (2023): 100381, https://doi.org/10.1016/j.ijchp.2023.100381.
9. Tatsuya Jitsuishi and Atsushi Yamaguchi, "Structural Connector Hub Properties of the Thalamus in Large-Scale Brain Networks: White Matter Structure as an Anatomical Basis," *NeuroImage* 317 (August 2025): 121333, https://doi.org/10.1016/j.neuroimage.2025.121333.
10. Yvette I. Sheline et al., "The Default Mode Network and Self-Referential Processes in Depression," *Proceedings of the National Academy of Sciences* 106, no. 6 (2009): 1942–47, https://doi.org/10.1073/pnas.0812686106.
11. Fabio Giommi et al., "The (In)Flexible Self: Psychopathology, Mindfulness, and Neuroscience," *International Journal of Clinical and Health Psychology* 23, no. 4 (2023): 100381, https://doi.org/10.1016/j.ijchp.2023.100381.
12. Jesus Montero-Marin et al., "School-Based Mindfulness Training in Early Adolescence: What Works, for Whom and How in the MYRIAD Trial?," *Evidence Based Mental Health* 25, no. 3 (2022): 117–24, https://doi.org/10.1136/ebmental-2022-300439.
13. Willoughby B. Britton, "Can Mindfulness Be Too Much of a Good Thing? The Value of a Middle Way," *Current Opinion in Psychology* 28 (August 2019): 159–65, https://doi.org/10.1016/j.copsyc.2018.12.011.
14. Nassim Nicholas Taleb, *Antifragile: Things That Gain from Disorder*, 1st edition (Random House, 2012).

Chapter 12: Be a Professional at Living Your Life

1. Tara O'Neill Hayes and Rosie Delk, "Understanding the Social Determinants of Health," September 3, 2018, https://www.americanactionforum.org/research/understanding-the-social-determinants-of-health/.
2. Mark Rose, "Anxiety Disorders" (Course #96182)," NetCE, Sacramento, California, 2022.
3. W. Timothy Gallwey, *The Inner Game of Tennis*, revised edition (Random House, 1997).
4. Alvaro Pascual-Leone et al., "Modulation of Cortical Motor Output Maps During Development of Implicit and Explicit Knowledge," *Science* 263, no. 5151 (1994): 1287–89, https://doi.org/10.1126/science.8122113.
5. E. G. Hall and E. S. Erffmeyer, "The Effect of Visuo-Motor Behavior Rehearsal with Videotaped Modeling on Free Throw Accuracy of Intercollegiate Female Basketball Players," *Journal of Sport Psychology* 5, no. 3 (n.d.): 343–46.
6. Alessandra Mancini and Francesco Mancini, "Rescripting Memory, Redefining the Self: A Meta-Emotional Perspective on the Hypothesized Mechanism(s) of Imagery Rescripting," *Frontiers in Psychology* 9 (April 2018): 581, https://doi.org/10.3389/fpsyg.2018.00581.
7. Lauren Stavropoulos et al., "Self-Guided Imagery Rescripting for Worry Images: A Preliminary Experimental Investigation," *Journal of Clinical Psychology* 80, no. 6 (2024): 1213–30, https://doi.org/10.1002/jclp.23660.
8. Lauren Doan et al., "Feasibility, Acceptability, Patient Experience, and Preliminary Efficacy of a Virtual Reality Guided Imagery Intervention for Chronic Pain," *Frontiers in Digital Health* 7 (June 2025): 1505861, https://doi.org/10.3389/fdgth.2025.1505861.
9. Robert Frost, "A Servant to Servants," Henry Holt and Company, 1915.
10. David Z. Hambrick et al., "Is the Deliberate Practice View Defensible? A Review of Evidence and Discussion of Issues," *Frontiers in Psychology* 11 (August 2020): 1134, https://doi.org/10.3389/fpsyg.2020.01134.
11. Steven W. Cole, "Human Social Genomics," *PLoS Genetics* 10, no. 8 (2014): e1004601, https://doi.org/10.1371/journal.pgen.1004601.
12. Bernie S. Siegel, *Love, Medicine, & Miracles: Lessons Learned About Self-Healing from a Surgeon's Experience with Exceptional Patients*, 1st Perennial Library (Harper & Row, 1988).

Epilogue

1. Rodney King, "Transcript of Rodney King's Statement," *Tampa Bay Times*, May 2, 1992, https://www.tampabay.com/archive/1992/05/02/transcript-of-rodney-king-s-statement/.

Index

Note: Page numbers in *italics* indicate figures.

D

About the Author

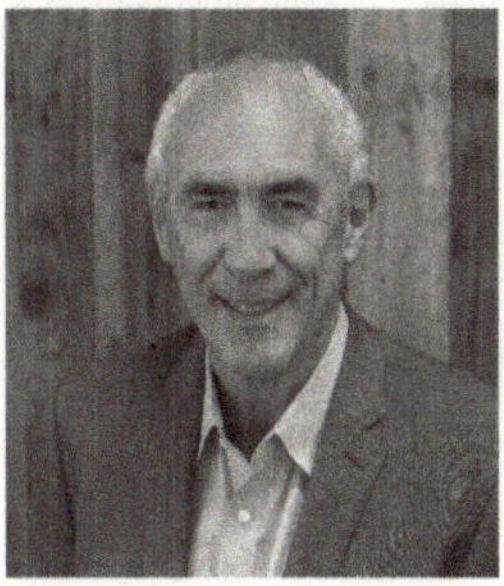

Clayton J. Mitchell Photography

For over three decades, Dr. David Hanscom practiced as an orthopedic complex spine surgeon in Seattle, Washington, and Sun Valley, Idaho. He later left his surgical practice to devote himself fully to education and advocacy. His work now spans books, blogs, podcasts, and lectures, including appearances on *Good Morning America*, *Dr. Oz*, CBS Radio, and *Psychology Today*. He is the author of *Back in Control: A Surgeon's Roadmap Out of Chronic Pain* and *Do You Really Need Spine Surgery? Take Control with a Surgeon's Advice*.

Dr. Hanscom is also a cofounder of the informal Dynamic Healing scientific study group, which dives into the deep data regarding chronic illness. His mission is to help people escape the abyss of pain and repetitive unwanted thoughts, reclaim their lives, and embrace the gift of consciousness by connecting cutting-edge science with lived human experience. His work and virtual courses can be found at backincontrol.com and thedocjourney.com.